RUSTY'S WAR
A BATTLE OF THE MIND

Michael Gordon Bennett

Bennett Global Entertainment Publishing
LAS VEGAS, NV

BGE Bennett
Global
Entertainment

PUBLISHING DIVISION

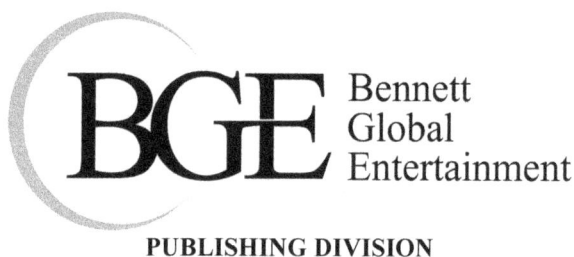

Bennett Global Entertainment Publishing
10695 Dean Martin Dr., #1027
Las Vegas, NV 89141
www.michaelgordonbennett.com

Cover Design: Kenleederdesign.co.uk

Rusty War: A Battle of the Mind. -- 1st ed.
ISBN 978-0-9864162-2-4

A portion of the proceeds from this book and speaking engagements will be donated to Alzheimer's care and research.

ii

To my mother, Anita, I've wept often knowing most of what makes us human, in you, has faded to black thanks to the ravages of Alzheimer's. I will always cherish our special bond and fight everyday to provide you comfort. I love you…Michael

Author's Note

Alzheimer's is the sixth leading cause of death in the United States. At the time of my mother's diagnosis, I thought nothing of the disease, thinking it more a byproduct of the natural aging process. In the words of Dale Carnegie, any man can make mistakes, but only an idiot persists in his error.

First, let me dispel the assumption, that Alzheimer's is part of the natural aging process; it's NOT. People in their mid-forties have been diagnosed with what we now know to be pre-Alzheimer's, often referred to as early onset Alzheimer's.

What is Alzheimer's? It's a devastating degenerative brain disorder that devours the memory and control of certain bodily functions.

By the time I became knowledgeable about the disease, my mother had passed through the early mild stage of Alzheimer's into the moderate level; complete with a host of behavioral changes including: paranoia, hallucinations, agitation, irrational fear and sixty years of lost memories.

Globally, an estimated 44 million people suffer from Alzheimer's. As of 2016, my mother is one of 5.4 million Americans suffering a slow death of the mind. Mom's diagnosis came three years before I wrote this book. Even with this discovery, she managed to spend significant portions of the next two-and-a-half years living alone, before dangers to self and others forced a change.

When she moved in, it didn't take long to realize Mom had a different symphony playing in her head, its rhythm so disjointed, you couldn't understand the melody or the lyrics.

Alzheimer's changed our lives, and hers, in unfathomable ways, as this insidious disease marched through Mom's brain destroying the synapses and neurons, and with it normal cognitive function. Her cerebral decline is so pronounced, things like speaking, eating, and bathing present monumental challenges, that when successful are worth celebrating.

Mom doesn't remember anything past childhood, in fact, most days she doesn't remember what happened five minutes ago. She experiences intermittent communication problems, unable to put coherent thoughts together. A lifetime of lost memories tells only part of the story.

Our future is likely to include; incontinence, feeding problems, the inability to talk and walk, soiled bed linens, adult diapers, and a host of illnesses that could kill her, all related to Alzheimer's.

In addition to the physical and mental decline, this disease is a hungry beast with a voracious appetite for money. The cost of care for the average American family is so prohibitive, entire savings for both the sufferer, and family care provider have been wiped out.

Homes have been foreclosed upon. Families have filed for bankruptcy.

U.S. caregivers have lost tens of billions of dollars in potential income to stay at home and tend to their suffering relative. Hundreds of thousands of caregivers have sacrificed their own health, often, going hungry, to save money to feed a loved one.

According to the Alzheimer's Association, the cost of caring for U.S. patients, in 2016, is $236 billion annually and climbing rapidly.

Fifteen million Americans provide unpaid care. That's an estimated 18.1 billion hours of informal work contributing $221.3 billion annually to the economy. The cost of care combined with lost family income will exceed a trillion dollars annually within two decades.

Diagnosed cases in America are projected to reach 13.8 million by 2050. Alzheimer's is America's fastest growing and least funded disease, in terms of both committed research dollars and care, and is by far the most costly to manage.

The National Institutes of Health (NIH) spends $6 billion a year on cancer research, $4 billion on heart disease and $3 billion on HIV/AIDS. By comparison, NIH spends a paltry $480 million on Alzheimer's.

Several studies point to family member caregivers supplementing the sufferers' income up to $100,000 annually---after the dementia patient has exhausted their savings, second mortgages, Medicaid, if they qualify, and long-term care insurance, if they're fortunate to find a good policy, and start early enough in life to make it a viable option.

What's being done about these runaway costs? Not much. Our profit-driven health care system doesn't adequately address America's most costly disease. The system exacerbates the experiences of our families, frustrating those desperately seeking financial help.

Organizations like the Alzheimer's Association, Helping Hands, here in Las Vegas, and Hilarity for Charity, founded by writer/actor Lauren Miller Rogen, and husband, actor Seth Rogen, provide financial vouchers to help offset care costs. But their funds are limited and depend primarily on donations.

Hilarity for Charity focuses on in-home care, and to date has provided over 56,000 hours of respite care across the United States and Canada.

The Alzheimer's Association and Helping Hands provide $500 to $1,000 vouchers, to be used for a combination of in-home or out-of-home care from licensed and approved providers.

These groups and others, such as NIH, and the scientific community are blowing the whistle and pounding on doors of our political leaders to do more, but they can't do it alone. Make no mistake, this isn't a looming crisis, the crisis is already here and they need our help.

Our story is intensely personal, many parts embarrassing beyond belief. But we felt compelled to shine a bright spotlight on our experiences with this debilitating disease, and its destructive path through our lives.

I plan to donate a portion of book sales and future speaking engagements to both Alzheimer's research and care. Additionally, I intend to find my own voice in myriad ways to raise awareness, this book being a first step. I will use the remainder of proceeds for my mother's care. While I could be selfish and can keep all the profits for Mom's sustenance and comfort, she would insist we help those who suffer like her and the less fortunate. In keeping with her spirit, I honor Mom's commitment to others.

Healthy Brain   Severe AD

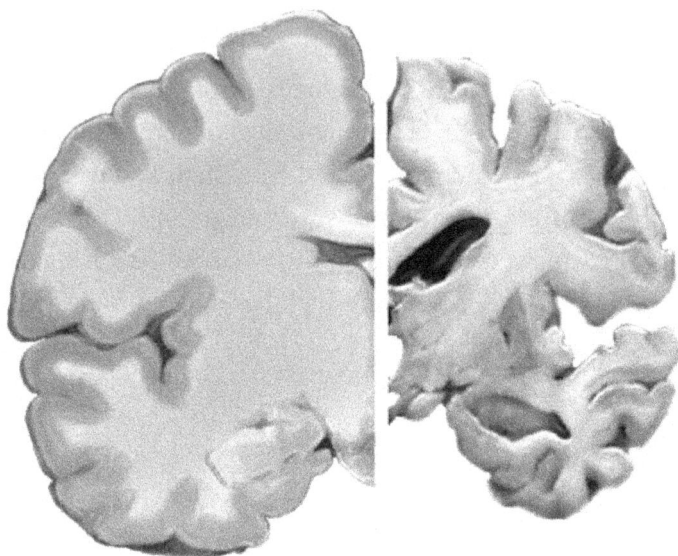

From the National Institute of Health

Contents

PROLOGUE

Hi, my name is Rusty, that cute little guy on the front cover. Yeah, yeah, save the wiener jokes. We dachshund's have a deep bark that sounds like it comes from a Rottweiler, and we use it liberally and without provocation in many instances. Our short stubby legs and barrel chest combined with fearlessness has intimidated the bravest of humans. I mean no harm, just know, I am the boss.

Dachshunds are intelligent, somewhat independent and playful. We can easily become a one-person dog, and that's exactly what happened to me.

I'm an eight-year-old who has been looking after an Alzheimer's victim for nearly four years. Between the barks, cries, and complex facial expressions, I developed my own language that helped me communicate with her. It worked so well in the beginning.

Then Alzheimer's claimed more and more of her brain. She no longer interprets my signals or anticipates my needs; and no matter how hard I try, I can't figure her out either.

When my owner brought me home, I was just eight weeks old; a scared little bundle of joy that rarely left

1

my two-legged mommy's side. We dachshunds love to cuddle. I'd curl up next to her at every opportunity, pushing myself to feel the warmth of her thigh.

When I became a little more sure-footed, I'd climb onto the sofa pillows that supported her back. She'd tilt her head back resting on me as if I were an elongated heated pillow. We were in heaven.

It took awhile to house train me. I can be downright stubborn. Besides, what was in it for me? I could go anywhere---the floor, the carpet, the backyard, I really didn't care. Someone else cleaned up the mess. My owner exercised a great deal of patience, and eventually I got the memo, the treats weren't bad either.

When I arrived at my new home, there was another dog, a sixteen-year-old cocker spaniel named Bella. Bella was Mom's soul mate, but Bella's body had begun to fail. When I wanted to play, Bella simply laid down, her movements trapped by mild paralysis that would worsen over time. She was too frail to match my boundless energy. Bella was mercifully put to sleep that first year ending her unendurable suffering. Mommy cried like a baby as she called her son in California to relay the sad news. I smothered her with all the love my nine-pound body could muster, licking the tears from her face and hands.

In time, Mom and I became inseparable. When she left home for church, the grocery store, or Tai Chi, I hated the separation, crying loudly until I heard the noise of the garage door as it opened. My tail wagged violently in anxious anticipation. At times I got so excited I peed on the floor.

In eight years, she'd only left me overnight twice, otherwise, it was just me and Mom; my best friend. She read lots of books those first five years. Dachshunds are nosy by nature; pardon my warped sense of humor. I sniffed each book as if searching for contraband, before she'd snatch the book from under my nose. *"Can I read it now,"* she'd ask, voice dripping with playful sarcasm.

We watched television, napped, ate dinner together and, played. She often fed me her food, even though she knew better. That food tasted so much better than the dry concoction in my dish.

At bedtime, I slept on the pillow next to Mom's head, or under the covers at her feet. Occasionally, I'd hear a noise at night alerting her to possible intrusion. I'm certain my bark discouraged more than a few brave souls. This is my house; enter at your own risk.

As you might have guessed, I'm spoiled. Mom obsessed over my care with monthly trips to the groomer. Some daring vet poked me with needles about once a year. I hated the vet, but tolerated their presence because mommy told me the temporary pain was for my own good.

Without warning, things began to change. While she always spoke to me like a human, the conversations were longer and more intense, often incoherent. I'd turn my head from side to side, brow furrowed, trying to make sense of it all, but decided to just lend an ear.

Mom stopped attending church and Tai Chi class; in fact, she seldom left the house, except a weekly trip to the grocery store. She quit answering the phone unless it was one of her three kids. Her withdrawal from society had begun.

Her daughter moved in and brought me two four-legged playmates. Mom took doggy care seriously. The arrival of my two companions actually masked what should have been obvious. She began to act confused. Then the pain of severe gastrointestinal problems robbed her of movement for about two hours each and everyday. All I could do was sit and watch as she clutched her stomach, rocking back and forth until the pain subsided.

Her son moved to Las Vegas, and quickly noticed the winds of change in his mother's behavior. It wasn't long before he started taking her to doctors all across the Las Vegas Valley. The gastrointestinal problems, on the surface, appeared to be the more pressing malady, as you could actually see the pain that wrecked her body.

Then she started to complain about her memory. *"I can't remember anything,"* she often told Michael, except me of course. At first, he thought it was a function of aging. Michael soon realized something far more sinister afoot.

She had no fewer than ten appointments a month for an entire summer. It was stomach specialist one day, memory doctors the next, all mixed in with scans, MRI's and enough blood tests to satisfy a flock of vampires. Michael didn't work that summer, so occupied with her care.

I became even more protective, probably to the point of irritation, but she never complained. In fact, she embraced my love, as I became the only true constant in her life.

In April 2013, the middle of my fifth year with Mom, Michael had taken over everything from paying her bills to medical decisions. It was that month she would be diagnosed with Alzheimer's. The news devastated Michael, but Mom didn't understand what any of it meant, happy to have Michael around to assume control of the confusing parts of her life.

The only thing she seemed to remember was overfeeding us dogs. I ate so much the next two years my excessive weight gain could have easily killed me. Despite her children's demands to get Mom to pull back on the food, she steadfastly refused. But her refusal wasn't one of contempt or disregard for my wellbeing, she simply couldn't remember having fed me.

Mom continued her withdrawal, often leaving the house in total darkness except the light flickering from the television set, or the backyard porch light, where she left the door open for us pooches to relieve ourselves. It didn't matter if it was 110 degrees outside, or ten, that door remained open.

When the doorbell rang, it startled her, the fear palpable. On Halloween night, as the neighborhood kids ran around hollering "trick or treat," Mom summoned

Michael to protect her from the local elementary school kids that populated our suburban home.

On the Fourth of July, the exploding fireworks left both of us trembling in fear. Michael, once again, came to the rescue.

Mom's interpretation of my signals worsened. I cried when I couldn't sit next to her, but she thought I was in pain. She called Michael every time I whimpered, often having him drive two hours, just to satisfy her paranoia. I licked his hand as he examined my body. He quickly realized the problems were in Mom's head.

When my little stomach was full and I refused to eat, she insisted Michael take me to the vet. It never occurred to her that I couldn't eat anymore. It got so bad, she would take food from my plate, and put it on the bedspread, or under the sheets at night, thinking the sight and smell would compel me to consume more. I seldom touched those crumbs, leaving the bed a gritty mess.

Mom would awaken in the middle of the night, sneak into the kitchen, and bring more food into her bedroom and sit in front of me eating. *"You want to eat something pumpkin,"* one of her nicknames for me. She proceeded to feed me bananas, soup, crackers, and pieces of her leftover sandwich. I didn't have enough sense to say no.

By morning, most of my partially undigested food would be in a messy pile on the carpet, Mom clueless as to its origin.

Nearly three years after the Alzheimer's diagnosis, life took an abrupt turn for the worse. An intervention arrived under terrible circumstances. Here is the story of mommy and me as written by my big brother, Michael.

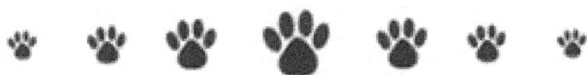

ACT 1

*"I think until you see Alzheimer's firsthand, it's kind of hard
to conceive how brutal it really is."*
Seth Rogen, Actor

CHAPTER ONE

Meltdown

"She's going to kill me," the hushed voice said, dripping in unrelenting fear. "Who, who is going to kill you?" "She's going to kill me, please come," the voice repeated, it's tone so grave I thought death was imminent. The voice remained frozen in place, hiding behind a rack of clothes inside a walk-in closet.

A journey that should have taken three quarters of an hour, took a mere thirty minutes as I sped north on Interstate 15 at ninety-miles-per-hour. We arrived to a phalanx of police cars, a fire truck and one ambulance blocking the driveway. Red and blue lights flashed repeatedly. Loud sounds of police radios ruined the peace and tranquility of this quiet suburban community, where kids normally played in the streets without fear, until well after dark. Neighbors peered from windows in all directions: one of them had called the police.

It was late February, approximately two hours after sunset. Police quickly verified my identity and began a detailed explanation of their need to rush to the scene. One of your mom's neighbors called 9-1-1, the officer told me.

They heard screaming, cussing and, what they later found out to be dishes and other glassware smashed against walls throughout the house. The dogs were going berserk as if the noise might have come from an intruder.

When we arrived, the lead officer at the scene said, they found this woman---the officer pointing towards a tall, thin woman, her face a deep crimson that I assumed came about in anger, standing nearby in handcuffs. She was screaming and throwing things around the house threatening to kill your mother. We asked her to tell us what happened and she just started on another incoherent tirade. We still don't know why she went after your mother.

Where did you find my mother? We searched the house and found her hiding in the closet. How did you coax Mom to come out? It took a few minutes, but if I had to guess, the officer said, she recognized our uniforms. As a former military spouse, Mom learned to respect any uniform, deeming its occupant to be friendly.

Mom hadn't spotted me yet. I could see from her interaction with police she operated in a state of total confusion. She was fully clothed, wrapped in a brown blanket, a defense against the cool night air. The temperature this early evening dipped into the low forties.

Other officers were engaged in a heated discussion with her caregiver, whose incoherent rants continued to pierce the night air, drowning out sounds emanating from the officer's squawk boxes. She screamed at the officers about something Mom did, or did not do, jerking against her handcuffs calling my mother a bitch. I flew off in the direction of this woman only to be restrained by an officer, no easy task given my size. The officers, on the other hand, exercised monumental restraint as she spat upon him.

After the quick debrief, I walked over to hug Mom. She looked at me for a brief moment, searching her memory for recognition, before she would allow an embrace. She had no clue what caused all the commotion, nor did she care.

She forgot all about Simone's meltdown; Alzheimer's took care of that. "Why are all these people at my house?" I chose not to explain, preferring to provide comfort and reassurance. Besides, I needed to calm my emotions, looking for an excuse to stay away from the woman charged with Mom's care.

Officers asked Mom a series of questions, before I told them about her memory. They gave me that "well that explains it look," Mom so completely unresponsive to their inquiries. All Mom could do was shrug her shoulders in defense against the unknowable.

Karen rushed home from work, breaking speed records like we had moments earlier. Prior to hiring a caregiver, Mom spent eight to ten hours a day, five days a week home alone. Her degenerative brain disorder made staying alone no longer tenable, and down right dangerous. Now I found myself questioning the meaning of dangerous.

As the police continued their investigation, my girlfriend played defense better than the newly crowned Super Bowl champion Denver Broncos, blocking my sister Karen's access to the care provider. Officers had just revealed to all of us that the caregiver reeked of alcohol and would be taken away.

This would be Mom's last night in her own home. After months of back and forth creating a workable plan for her care, we were back to square one.

I hoped the care provider solution would last just a little longer, allowing me enough time to land on my feet after launching a new business. My intent had always been to have Mom live with me under the care of a full time nurse, assuming my income would improve enough to make it affordable. I traveled for a living, making supervision an absolute necessity.

Her rapidly deteriorating memory, and the immediate loss of that caregiver sent my heart rate soaring. I found it difficult in that moment to breathe normally. Mom's cognitive function had already diminished to a more advanced stage of Alzheimer's and I totally missed the announcement.

I visited her several times a month, taking her to every doctor's appointment, the movies, and out for dinner, yet I missed every sign of decline, the procession so subtle. Standing in the cool night air, observing

Mom's diminished mental capacity punctured my psyche, and it hurt.

As a precaution, and need for an alternative plan, we spent the prior month touring traditional assisted living facilities. Each had a memory care wing, but I didn't think Mom required that level of care. My immediate observations proved how terribly wrong I'd been.

Mom still had life in that body. I was determined to squeeze every once of enjoyment out of it before I'd even consider a memory care facility. Denial based on love is powerful.

I always thought I had more time to make these life-altering decisions, the love for my mother trumping any semblance of my common sense. That love provided me an excuse to ignore reality. I was already in a race against a known enemy with its own timetable for destruction. I hadn't prepared for battle.

Karen initially resisted any discussion of assisted living, believing she could still care for Mom, which in hindsight wasn't feasible. Working forty to fifty hours a week, then coming home to a second fulltime job, left my poor sister exhausted, frustrated and angry. Mom's care dominated her life, as was the growing annoyance at being unable to communicate with Mom's confusion and rapidly expanding paranoia and incoherence.

* * *

The ambulance and police left after nearly ninety minutes. "Mom, you're coming to stay with me tonight." "Is Rusty coming?" "Of course, I wouldn't leave your buddy." Mom smiled. We packed a single suitcase, grabbed her four-legged companion of eight years, and drove to our two-bedroom apartment on the south side of Las Vegas.

Mom marveled at the bright lights of the Las Vegas Strip whizzing by at seventy miles-per-hour on Interstate 15. Looking at her, it was obvious she thought this was new territory, not the city she'd lived in for the past ten years.

My girlfriend and I were quiet. The freedom to come and go as we pleased had just come to an abrupt halt. I felt detached from the car, floating on a higher plane, lost in deep thought---what now?

I occasionally looked over at Mom. She had this empty gaze, something I now call the "Alzheimer's Stare." The woman I called mom all these years, while physically still very much with us, had disappeared. No longer would I be able to ask for advice, or confide in her. It simply never crossed my mind that one day I would be my mother's parent. My eyes moistened as I fought to keep my vision clear long enough to get us home.

For the next four nights, Mom slept on our living room sofa, until I could clear out the second bedroom, which had previously been my home office. She thoroughly enjoyed being the center of attention.

Our apartment was no place for three people and a dog. I questioned everything, reflecting on all the mistakes I made thinking time was an ally not an enemy.

Could we care for Mom? Where would the money come from? I sunk every dime of my savings into a new business. We were in serious trouble with no long-term solution readily apparent.

Then I began to worry my girlfriend would leave. She certainly hadn't planned on caring for an Alzheimer's patient when we met three years earlier. It would require a tremendous sacrifice to a man she had yet to marry.

To her credit, she stayed. It wasn't without its challenges. One advantage she had that I didn't, it was my mom, not hers. My emotional attachment made me hesitant at times to seize control of the situation. That hesitation would be reflected in several poor decisions I made over the next few months, as I rushed to catch up to a disease I knew so little about.

CHAPTER TWO

Retirement

Eleven years earlier --- Sierra Vista, AZ: I listened intently as Mom told the gathering of soon to be former co-workers, her reasons for retirement, at a celebration of her service at a local restaurant.

She gave thirty-five years of her life to the Army Air Force Exchange Service. From Maine to Florida to Colorado Mom managed to continue her career on each of Dad's military reassignments.

After their divorce in the early eighties, she forged ahead: career advancements coming rapidly, despite having nothing more than a high school education. Mom's career path eventually carried her to a supervisory position at Ft. Huachuca, an Army post southeast of Tucson, about fifteen miles from the Mexican border. It was the former home of the Buffalo Soldiers---the old Negro Calvary units of the post Civil

War era. She told the audience it was simply *"time to go home to her family."*

Deep down, I knew there was more; call it a son's intuition. While many consider sixty-five-years-old, retirement age, she enjoyed her work, and had no physical limitations that would have prevented her from continuing for another five years. Maybe she really was tired, but I was highly suspicious.

As Mom continued, I noted the sadness in her hazel eyes, those eyes, the envy of everyone she ever came in contact with, the look so captivating, against her light chocolate skin. Despite her age, her skin was wrinkle free, looking much like she did in her thirties, absent the gray hair.

She looked down several times, choking back tears, the lump in her throat forcing a momentary pause in her remarks. Mom hated public speaking, the fact she stood this long was a monumental endeavor. These people were family, arguably just as meaningful to Mom as her biological one. My clairvoyance would eventually be proven correct, but today wasn't the day to push the envelope. Mom needed to enjoy the adulation she so richly deserved.

Just like that it was all over. Some friendships would be maintained for a few years, but like most military families, you simply moved on to the next phase of your life. If you see one another again, that's great, but we all understood, life goes on, not an existence for the faint of heart. This time it would be different. Mom officially retired. No more new assignments and new military families to befriend.

For Mom, the military was all she'd known since high school graduation. She most certainly didn't take the decision to retire lightly. Mom would now be alone for long periods of time. All her three of her children and two grandchildren lived on the west coast, but we were busy with life. None of us stopped to think about incorporating Mom into our plans, beyond her frequent visits. Her retirement had been so abrupt, at least to us, we never stopped our train long enough to take on another passenger. Within a few years, she would come to dominate my life like no one previously---the train had come to a full stop.

I returned to my California home after her retirement ceremony obsessed with thoughts of the lonely life she led after divorce, now further exacerbated by retirement. She never remarried. The will was there, but Mom is such an introvert, it would have taken the gift of a thousand extroverts to approach her for a simple coffee date---somebody with the bold confidence to pull this wonderful sweet woman out of her shell. She could blend in and shy away better than anybody I've ever known. Now her work family would soon disappear.

I remained convinced some internal voice pushed her towards retirement. I spent Christmas with Mom at her Sierra Vista home and helped prepare the house for sale. She decided to move to Las Vegas to be nearer her children and grandchildren. One of my sister's lived in Vegas, the other, near me in Southern California.

I managed to get my mother talking, no easy task. Our conversation lasted several hours, while I worked around the house fixing plumbing; painting, replacing light bulbs and performing light yard work. Desert landscaping didn't require much effort, allowing me plenty of time to engage her in conversation. She mentioned her memory, jokingly, dismissing it as a factor of aging. I left for California after the New Years holiday, no closer to the truth about the real reason she retired.

It was 2 a.m. The streets outside my Los Angeles apartment were quiet. I rose from bed and walked to the kitchen for a glass of water. I sat staring at the other high rises in the area. The lights were mostly off at this hour. I had a vivid dream about retirement and death that startled me out of a deep slumber. Something just didn't add up. She'd retired abruptly. Mom was not impulsive by nature; in fact, she made decisions so slow at times it annoyed me.

What could make her act so fast? As if the heavens opened up to provide an answer, I realized it had something to do with memory. The frequent jokes about memory were actually clues. While simply forgetting her keys wouldn't raise alarm bells, my other observations began to establish a pattern. Forgetting obvious facts of her immediate past, her inability to read a traditional clock, relying more on digital versions, fumbling for words, and more.

I called later that morning. "Mom did you retire because you believe you're losing your memory?" She was insulted I would even broach the subject, letting me know, as only she could, to butt out of her business.

Mom never spoke to me in such a manner, even during my childhood. I'd always been her confidant, even more so than her husband, my father, who she divorced decades earlier because of his alcoholism. When she needed an outlet for her emotions during my teenaged years, it was me she chose to share her burdens at the risk of upsetting my father. It was a tremendous responsibility for any teenager, but I had enough sense to never betray her faith in me and kept my mouth shut. Besides, I understood. Dad's ugly behavior was either directed at mom or me, until one of my sister's made the colossal mistake of challenging his authority, which occurred frequently now as he spent more and more of his time away from home drinking.

I stayed away from home in high school to avoid confrontation with Dad. Mom had no such luxury and endured a great deal of heartbreak and anguish until she summoned the courage to divorce him, largely at my urging.

What we didn't understand at the time; was Dad's irrational behavior and mood swings were a cry for help. He returned from Vietnam, with what we now know to be Post Traumatic Stress Disorder (PTSD). We'd never heard of PTSD until well after their divorce. Mom battled it all, suppressing her emotional wellbeing for the sake of us kids. To this day, I don't know how she survived.

Her reaction to my question about lost memory confirmed my suspicions. It would be another month before she revealed her secret; then swore me to secrecy. But she really hadn't admitted to anything truly alarming, other than temporary bouts of forgetfulness, certainly nothing out of the ordinary for a senior citizen. Yet, fear gripped her words with a certainty that caught my attention.

At the time of her admission, I didn't realize her mother had Alzheimer's, and her father would soon be diagnosed with dementia. In hindsight, I'm sure Mom already knew, and the revelation heightened her sense of awareness and insecurity. Her parents' were both in their late eighties at the time---Mom still in her mid-sixties. Was she experiencing true symptoms, sympathetic symptoms, or simply being proactive?

* * *

In April 2006, Mom closed on her new house in the greater Las Vegas area, and got on with living the life of a retiree. The single-story, three-bedroom, two-bath home would become her sanctuary until the night police arrived. I planned to stay a month to help her get acclimated. The timing was perfect. I recently divorced and needed to decompress. It would be three years before I made it back to California.

We started by finding Mom a church, a source of great comfort throughout her life. Her mother worked and led the choir at St James AME church, in Atlantic

City, for decades. Mom's grandparents' had also been members of that same church. Her family established a legacy at St. James that dated back to just after the turn of the twentieth century.

It took us almost a year, but we found a church to her liking. It helped that her best friend of thirty years from Colorado Springs, moved to the area, and joined the same church.

Mom planned her Sunday's in the fall around church and football. From 8 a.m. to 10 a.m., it was church. From 10 a.m. to 6 p.m., the NFL; then back to church from 7 p.m. to 9 p.m. for the children's ministry. If the Denver Broncos were on television, the outside world ceased to exist.

Monday night, it was more football, including all the pre-game shows. She was hooked on a sport I taught her during my high school years.

I would head to the basement of our Air Force Academy home, where we had a television lounge. At first, I sat alone, enjoying the solitude, and escape from our unhappy household---my focus on the game and the announcer's voice. Dad wasn't a big sports fan, except Baltimore Orioles baseball.

Mom would drift downstairs on occasion with a cup of coffee, sit quiet as a church mouse, and watch for a few minutes and disappear. A few weeks later, she would watch an entire quarter. One quarter became two, and before I knew it, I had a companion for an entire game, then two games. We would repeat the routine for Monday Night Football, just the two of us. Frank

Gifford, Howard Cosell, and "Dandy" Don Meredith became household names.

After a month of joining me in the basement, she started asking questions. *What's a first down? How many yards do you need to make a first down? How many downs are there? Why is a field goal worth three points? What's a screen pass? What's a tight end?* The questions were endless. Normally, I'd be upset when someone interrupted my game, but for some reason, I didn't mind answering. I guess it gave me a chance to show off. The more Mom asked, the more she got into the game, screaming at the television on occasion, in an outburst that startled even my hyper competitive spirit.

It was here she became a Denver Broncos fan. We had our own little friendly rivalry in those days, me being a huge supporter of the Pittsburgh Steelers. I had the upper hand back then, as the Steelers were in the midst of four Super Bowl wins in a six-year span.

How ironic the owner of her favorite football team, Pat Bowlen, would relinquish control of his team in 2014 thanks to Alzheimer's.

* * *

To Mom's credit, she realized she couldn't sit around the house all day and watch television without some form of exercise. She called around and found a place that offered Tai Chi classes. Why Tai Chi, I have no idea. She came home one day with a board she actually split in two, with what I was told was a beautifully executed punch. I didn't know they taught that in Tai Chi, I thought it was more about the movement. Tai Chi got her away from the house three days a week. Combined with church, that was a good amount of activity.

Mom and I started working on her new house. We contracted someone to build a patio cover. I painted every room in the house, nearly falling off the ladder on numerous occasions as I stretched to reach the top of her twelve-foot vaulted ceilings. We had custom blinds made. We hired a gardener to landscape the yard and bring in new trees. Helping her was just the therapy I needed. Never once did I reveal my own angst at my personal situation, taking a page from Mom's book, keeping my feelings to myself. Like mother like son.

Mom knew, without saying a word, I was suffering, but talking about it right then would have been futile, and she knew it---just let me work, I'll eventually land on my feet.

In those days, Mom paid all her own bills, meticulously accounting for every penny. Her checkbook had to balance, or she'd be on the phone with the bank until the issue could be resolved. Yelling at a banker about her missing pennies was must see television.

Mom became a news junkie, spending her days switching back and forth between CNN, FOX, and MSNBC. The 2008 presidential election cycle would be her first as a Nevada resident, and it didn't hurt that Barack Obama was running for his first term. Mom made sure we voted, and blasted my sister for not going to the polls, in a fit of anger that could blow the roof of her house, had she not been sitting in the backyard.

Mom had always been an avid reader, often two or three books a week. Since there wasn't a Barnes & Noble nearby, she would have books delivered. The UPS driver knew me by name. Whose reading all of these books, he asked one hot summer afternoon. Mom, I said, they are all trashy romance novels. We both laughed. Each time he stopped at the door, we chuckled at the contents of Mom's boxes, wondering how anyone could publish so much make believe filth. Once, he fled the house in a hurry as mom headed for the door to curse at both of us for teasing her about those books. Within a year, Mom purchased enough books to stock a small library.

Life was good for Mom. She did her own shopping, took care of her then 13-year-old cocker spaniel, Bella, and actually decided to get another dog three years later, a dachshund she named Rusty. Rusty was a quick study with an infectious personality. This charming little guy fit right in, taking control of Mom's emotions from the moment he sit foot in her house.

Mom would mention her memory about once a month in passing. She functioned on all cylinders, near as I could tell. Family visited often, adding to the picture in her mind of what retirement was supposed to represent.

I drove her to Cleveland, OH, once (she hates to fly) to spend a week with her aging parents'. It was during this trip, in 2008, that I discovered both her parents' had been diagnosed with dementia. I hadn't seen my grandparents' in six years, and wasn't prepared for their cerebral decline.

I entered their home hugging and kissing them as if life were normal. They acted like they knew me, but weren't certain, as each paused a little before returning my embrace.

Despite the disease, they both seemed in good spirits, thanks to the care of Mom's younger sister. Mom seemed to know about the dementia, but never mentioned it during our three-day drive. Maybe she didn't understand the disease, or thought it none of my business. Regardless of her intent, I was none too happy. I'd been blindsided. Mom had insisted on this trip like nothing before in her life, and needed me to make it happen. Now I knew why she was so adamant.

It wasn't until my aunt asked my grandmother if she recognized her only grandson that I realized she suffered from a disease I only knew by name.

My aunt proceeded to show them several photos of me prominently displayed in their apartment. My grandmother's face lit up like Times Square as she put the photo and the real live me together. I looked at my grandfather and noticed his recognition and reaction to my being there was noticeably quicker. "I know who you are," he said, smiling. He surprised me with that comment. Grandpop hadn't spoken a word since we entered their domain.

For the next week, I walked around on eggshells unsure what I should, and shouldn't do. How do you communicate with not one, but two Alzheimer's sufferers? Once again, my aunt stepped up and provided guidance.

Then my grandmother burst into the room shouting, "where's my boyfriend." She was referring to me. It took several minutes to convince her of my true identity. That was my first experience with a hallucination, yet from my grandmother's perspective, it was real.

I spent the remainder of our visit observing their behavior. My first conclusion, neither of them seemed to sleep. I woke every few hours to noise coming from their bedroom. I peeked through the open door and found my grandmother folding clothes. A few hours later she was in the closet removing clothes and refolding them. She seemed content as my grandfather sat and watched. They exchanged words once every ten minutes or so, then back to the expected peace and tranquility of 3 a.m. It was wash, rinse and repeat every night.

Their eighth floor two-bedroom apartment was fully furnished with a side view of Lake Erie from their balcony, a balcony I'm certain they never used. The large television was connected to security cameras at the building's entrance. Rather than watch a program, many nights, after my aunt returned home for the evening, they sat watching people enter and exit the building. I guess maybe it was the closes thing to their home in Atlantic City, where the family gathered on the patio after dinner, to take in the sights and sounds of the neighborhood.

My aunt cooked all their food, but it had been ingrained in my grandmother for decades to prepare the family meal---a memory that survived Alzheimer's. She tried to help, but my aunt limited those tasks to simple things that didn't require much thought, effort or a stove. My aunt always took the time to include my grandmother---it was a beautiful site to behold.

Only once did I see either of my grandparents' express, or, act out in anger, although I found out later, it happened more often than I was aware. My grandfather, who suffered from diabetes, refused to elevate his feet as the doctor instructed. He resisted every attempt my aunt tried, until he lashed out at her. A minute later she tried again. She knew he no longer remembered his initial flare-up and complied with her request. It's a lesson I would put to good use in a few years.

My grandmother loved to grocery shop. I escorted my grandmother, mother, and aunt to a grocery store in Euclid, OH, one early afternoon. Mom went one way, my aunt another, and my grandmother to the frozen food section in another aisle to examine ice cream. I kept a respectful distance from the person I thought would need my help the most---my grandmother.

She spotted me hovering nearby, turned, shaking her cane in my direction, and said, "Go on, I don't need anybody watching me." I smiled, inwardly of course, because that fierce independent spirit is what made my Granny, my Granny. Alzheimer's couldn't rob her of that independence; she would go down kicking and screaming.

The drive back to Vegas was quiet that first day. Mom loved to travel by car, so I decided to try a more southerly route back home, going around the Rockies, rather than drive over them like I'd done en route to Cleveland. We passed through Columbus, Indianapolis, crossed the Mighty Mississippi in St Louis and spent the first night in Springfield, MO. Not once did we talk about her parents' or the elephant in the room.

The second day took us through Tulsa, Oklahoma City, and the Texas panhandle where we reminisced about our one night stay in Amarillo back in 1974, when we transferred from Florida to Colorado Springs. It was here I asked Mom about her own memory. "I'm fine." She appeared to be in complete control, I just needed reassurance.

* * *

I stayed with Mom for another year. In June 2009, I decided to get on with my life and return to California and re-launch my now stagnant career. It happened to be the same day Michael Jackson died, so I stayed behind a few days to avoid the circus. My apartment sat in the middle of all the action.

For the next eighteen months, life was good for both of us. My career started to gain traction once again, and Mom continued to live the wonderful life of a retiree.

Twenty months later, we would be back in Cleveland for my grandmother's funeral.

When my grandfather was wheeled in for my Granny's service, the entire family gathered around to support our patriarch.

My little cousin (age 3 or 4) approached his wheel chair in one of the most touching moments I've ever witnessed. He smiled as only he could at the site of this precious little girl hugging him.

Then Mom approached. He didn't recognize her despite both my aunts' and uncle providing an assist. It's the second time I'd ever seen her cry. I grabbed her hand and escorted her to a seat in the church, but for some reason Mom didn't want to sit in the front row with the rest of her siblings. She preferred the comfort of Karen and me one row back.

When we approached the casket, Mom squeezed my hand hard, forcing blood from my fingertips. She mumbled a few words about a memory from childhood, reached out to touch her mother's hand as family members and friends sobbed loudly nearby. This was the first time I'd been to a funeral for a family member in my life. All I could think to do was keep Mom upright. My grieving would have to wait until later. The woman, so at peace in that casket was more than a loved one, she was our hero.

* * *

Forty days later we were back in Cleveland. My grandfather left to join his love of seventy-three-years. It was at my grandfather's funeral that I finally started to see outward signs of Mom's short-term memory fading. It's a moment I'd mentally prepared for, but prayed would never come. Relatives reminisced about my grandparents' and various other events from our past. "Nita, you remember when we...?" Mom didn't remember, but was too ashamed to speak honestly, just nodding her head. Mom already started withdrawing from her own family before the trip---not taking calls, or resisting attempts to connect with her own kids, me included. I didn't start connecting the dots until now.

Once back home, I vowed to call and visit more often. Eighteen months later Dad died. They were high school sweethearts, married for twenty-five years, but divorced for nearly thirty years. We started reminiscing, when Karen said something about Dad. Mom looked at me and reacted like Dad didn't exist, despite numerous photos on her fireplace mantle of all of us, including him. This was not a bitter reaction to divorce; she genuinely didn't remember having been married.

I mentioned the need for testing, given what I now knew about her parents'. What I didn't know at the time, she had been pleading with her primary care physician for over a year to provide a referral to the Lou Ruvo Brain Institute in Las Vegas. It was mother being mother, never one to reveal too much. She confirmed, that in the two years since my return to California, she truly started having issues with memory loss. The time to act had long since passed.

CHAPTER THREE

Diagnosis

C hristmas 2012 --- I returned to Las Vegas to celebrate the holiday with Mom. It was a low-key affair, like recent observances---just the two of us. One look at her, and I knew, without reservation, I needed to stay. Her mental deterioration so pronounced, I wondered if she had been sabotaged by some doctor and injected with a drug that sped up the effects of Alzheimer's. I remain astounded to this day, so little could happen in such a short space of time.

She struggled to balance her checkbook. Little things around the house that she would never ignore; now went undone---dusty furnishing, dirty floors, piles of laundry and more. When I asked her about the laundry, she simply acted as if those dirty clothes had no other home except the floor.

A week later, despite my best efforts, the place still looked like a tornado swept through the premises.

I took up the cause of helping Mom get a referral to the Brain Institute. It seemed ridiculous to have one of the foremost brain research centers in the world in her backyard, and not have access to their care and guidance. Together we became a thorn in the side of her primary care physician.

She recently signed a medical power of attorney granting me final authority for all decisions. Mom trusted my judgment, but more importantly, she needed assistance remembering events, doctor instructions, and deciphering explanations in terms she could comprehend.

After weeks of nonstop calls, Mom's doctor demanded she appear at her office, tired of our pestering for that coveted referral. I was already annoyed at the lengths we had just undertaken to get a simple return phone call. A receptionist, who treated my mother as an inferior person, further exacerbated my anger. How dare you talk to my mother that way, I thought to myself, while I listened on the other line. I suppressed my outrage to focus on the greater good, but I already knew this appointment wasn't going to end well.

When we arrived, the doctor attempted a rather cryptic memory exam that felt more like a psychiatric test. I could no longer censor my tongue. I became enraged, physically grabbing Mom, shoving her towards the front door, fearful my irritation would land me in a jail cell. That would be the last time we saw that doctor, who shall remain nameless for obvious reasons, but who no longer has a private practice.

We found a new primary care physician, and started the explanation and history process all over again. Like her previous doctor, she was unconvinced Mom had any memory loss, thinking it more the rants of an old woman, seventy-two at the time.

Once again, we sought, and found a new primary care physician. This doctor proved more attentive to Mom's concerns. She sat and listened as we started to describe her experiences of the previous two plus years, and her inability to focus any longer. I added to Mom's lapse in recall as the doctor took copious notes. We were fortunate her new doctor had seen dementia before.

Despite our success at finally finding this gem of a physician, I remained dumbfounded so many doctors knew so little about Alzheimer's. I assumed communication with a patient to be a vital tool in their arsenal to provide quality care. As I was about to discover, communicating with the medical profession stood as a monumental challenge. I continually find myself explaining Mom's condition, and why, at times she is so unresponsive.

After nearly three years, we finally received our coveted referral, including a phone call from Mom's new primary care physician in advance of her first appointment.

The first appointment, in late February 2013, took an hour. I regurgitated for the umpteenth time, Mom's complete medical history dating back to my childhood. I had it all committed to memory, including dates. The doctor typed feverishly into his computer, astounded at my total recall. I knew her medical history better than my own.

The doctor immediately expressed his alarm at the copious amounts of Pepto Bismal Mom consumed on a daily basis. The doctor was so frightened by her admission, that he stopped the interview process, and began a clinical explanation of the harmful effects of Pepto Bismal on the brain. Mom understood none of it, but I hung on every word, absorbing the seriousness of the doctor's dire message.

Mom had her gallbladder removed in the fall of 2000. Since its removal, she suffered chronic bloating and gastrointestinal pains that were severe at times, leaving her short of breath, with accelerated blood pressure--- once measured during an attack at 162/70, well into stage two hypertension. These attacks typically lasted less than an hour.

Two specialists later, not to mention tens of thousands of dollars in exams, scans, tests, and evaluations, along with numerous emergency room visits---doctors found nothing, claiming she was really healthy, especially for someone her age.

Mom came to depend on Pepto Bismal like a junkie on heroin in her desperation for relief. The doctor explained how Pepto Bismal contained an ingredient called bismuth that blocked the body's absorption of protein, a vital nutrient for healthy brain function.

The doctor said, "stop Pepto Bismal now," in a voice so disturbing, it sounded like a command from God. I rose from my chair, excused myself for the moment under the guise I had to use the restroom, walked to the lobby and called Karen. I demanded she remove all Pepto Bismal from the house before we got home. My sister found four big bottles of the pink stuff hidden all over the house---many unopened. I found a few more when we returned.

A few years later, I saw a report on *Good Morning America* discussing the harmful effects of Pepto Bismal on the brain, and how it contributed to dementia. It didn't help that Mom completely disregarded the warning label that discussed short-term consumption---if symptoms persist please consult your physician. Mom ignored the warning because not a single physician provided her with any relief.

A week later we were back at the Cleveland Clinic for a two-hour evaluation. Mom answered questions, did a series of oral and written exams, and whatever else they do to test cognition that didn't require needles and scans.

I sat in the lobby reading literature about the clinic and the latest in advanced Alzheimer's research. While I was happy so many of the world's best minds were actively seeking a cure, nothing I read suggested they were close.

Another week elapsed before our return, this time for blood work, scans and an MRI. By now, I was fairly certain Mom had some form of dementia. The severity had yet to be determined.

April 4, 2013, all test results had been compiled into a neat report that her doctor was about to share. I sat in nervous anticipation. Mom remained motionless, unsure why she'd been called back to this place again.

What happened next, I still haven't recovered from nearly four years later. The imagery that lie before me seared into my subconscious tormenting my psyche--- that gray, rotted look of cauliflower representing parts of my mother's dead brain cells. The reduction in brain size rendered me speechless. Even a faux neurologist like myself knew those synapses no longer fired.

On the wall next to the lighted board that held my mom's MRI results, were several photos of a healthy brain. The contrast played like a cruel joke.

The doctor continued his explanation for what seemed like an eternity, but in reality lasted just a few minutes. I sat silently, listening, as the doctor tried to soften the blow. I glanced at Mom. She had that befuddled and confused countenance, unsure what any of this meant. We fought for three years to get a diagnosis, and it had all boiled down to this one-hour appointment.

The doctor continually grabbed Mom's hands, stroking them ever so gently, in a calm reassuring voice. Mom had yet to grasp the gravity of the situation and wondered why the doctor spoke to her so tenderly, like maybe he was planning to ask her out on a date. This doctor was a true professional and it showed in how he delivered the devastating news.

Mom was never one to comprehend even basic scientific knowledge, trusting the medical expert to tell her what to do in layman's terms. It was an unfortunate consequence of lack of a more advanced education, and our military background, where we are essentially taught to follow orders and trust superiors. After my combined twenty-eight years as a military brat and a veteran, it took me a couple of years to break the old habit of blind trust---a lesson mother never learned.

The doctor continued his exhaustive explanation, taking all the appropriate pauses to make sure I understood, and allow me to ask questions. My most pressing question at the time, "how far along is she?" I asked a second question about life expectancy, and a third about behavioral changes I should expect and when.

Based on their assessment, Mom had mild Alzheimer's. But the degenerative nature of this disease meant this would be the best mom in terms of cognition and brain function I would see ever again.

"Some patients live five years after diagnosis, others for twenty," the doctor said, "each is different." He couldn't be more definitive.

As for behavioral changes, we discussed aggression, agitation, confusion, and depression. He stopped and looked at Mom, "Anita are you depressed?" She gave an emphatic no, but I wondered if she knew what the word depression meant. Mom shot me that look of confusion that I'd come to recognize when she didn't understand something.

We talked about repetition and sleeplessness. Mom never slept for long periods of time, so I didn't pay much attention to this issue at first, having forgotten what I observed at my grandparents' home a few years earlier.

We left the doctor's office, with an appointment for two weeks later to discuss treatments and ways to cope, but not before the doctor suggested I start seeking support groups. The idea of a support group seemed bizarre at the time, showing my true naiveté. Mom needed help, not me. His admonition to join a support group went in one ear and right out the other---a gross error in judgment I'd come to regret later. At the time, I was more focused on how I would explain all of this to my dear mother.

What led us to the Cleveland Clinic in the first place was Mom's dogged determination to get to the bottom of her foggy memory. In the irony of all ironies, it had taken so long to reach this point in our quest for knowledge, that Mom no longer had the ability to comprehend the results, how sad.

As I expected on the ride home, she asked, *"What the hell was that all about?"* I swallowed hard for a moment knowing I needed to be delicate. She didn't understand terms like degenerative disease, and clinical explanations like plaques, tangles and neurons. I distilled this medical and scientific jargon into easy to digest terms, leaving out all the gory details.

Once I finished my simplistic explanation, a river of tears cascaded down her face dampening her light blue shirt. I took a hand off the steering wheel at the next red light, and grabbed her hand. Mom shook uncontrollably, she knew, without saying a word the curtain was about to close on her past. My hand remained on hers until I pulled the blue Toyota Yaris into the garage.

Rusty greeted us at the door with his normal puppy-like exuberance. It took about a minute before he realized something was amiss. He sat quietly while I escorted Mom to the sofa. I opened the backdoor for Rusty, but he refused to leave, choosing instead, to jump on the sofa to sit on her lap. He licked the very hand I had been holding ever so lovingly. His life too had just changed and I believe he sensed the inevitable.

We sat in silence for hours, me afraid to utter a single word for fear of upsetting her further. Mom turned on the television for a distraction. We started with news, but she was in no mood for serious commentary. After several moments of channel surfing, she settled on *Family Feud*, a program that would play a key role in her life as the destruction of her brain progressed.

I left for home well after dark, my mind on a teeter-totter of emotions---profound sadness one moment, the monumental task that laid ahead, the next. I had to start preparing for the inevitable. I'd seen the Devil's Disease from a distance, but I still didn't know the scope of my aunt's care and all she had endured on a daily basis.

Other than alerting my sisters', I kept my immediate thoughts to myself for months.

Shortly after diagnosis, we held a family reunion in Las Vegas. I, more than anyone, was thankful, knowing full well had it been any other place, Mom wouldn't attend, or I'd have to drive her across country. I also realized this would probably be the last time she would see, or even remember most of those in attendance. When we spoke to Mom about the upcoming reunion her reaction was rather blasé. She didn't care, content to remain locked inside the recesses of a mind she no longer controlled.

During our evening dinner, my cousins' and me took turns presenting awards and plaques to the patriarchs and matriarchs of our family, primarily our parents'. As I called Mom to the podium, her vacant stare told a story---one of complete detachment.

I read the following words from the plaque my sisters' and me presented to our mother.

A mother's love is never ending,
It never judges,
It never discriminates,
It's always there in your heart, where you'll find a
mother's love

With devotion and love
Your children,

Michael, Karen & Amanda

After I finished, the crowd stood in applause, Mom, on the other hand had no reaction, her time in the spotlight had come to a merciful end. If she were able to internalize those words, or comprehend their meaning, it never showed.

Mom participated little in the night's activities, preferring to sit silently at the round table near the front of the room with her brother and sisters'. She didn't initiate a single discussion. When others spoke to her, or gave their Aunt Nita a hug, she was cordial, more of her enduring politeness than any acknowledgment of the moment.

Someone took a great picture of the two of us. Looking at the photo months later, it proved to be a lasting forecast of the future. I can no longer look at that photo; the daze, the emptiness so strong it defies description.

The only moment of recognition for Mom that entire evening occurred when the music started. At first, some cousins and my youngest aunt, a professional singer, did a little karaoke. Mom enjoyed the moment, but didn't come into her element until the soundtrack was allowed to play without familial accompaniment. Mom danced violently in her seat, giving the poor strings on her chair a monumental stress test. She snapped her fingers and sang along loudly to the smorgasbord of tunes from the 1950s, 60s, and 70s. We were all delighted to see how engaged she'd become.

Mom had yet to reveal her diagnosis to family, but I think they knew. I actually broke the news to her siblings within the month, enduring the wrath of an aunt for not spilling the beans sooner. It's the first time I ever violated Mom's privacy, but I thought they should know. I remain unrepentant in my revelation to her family.

CHAPTER FOUR

Immediate Aftermath

The diagnosis was devastating. Alzheimer's creates the environment for a slow agonizing death. The thought that I could lose Mom to such an ugly disease overwhelmed all other thoughts and actions for days. My mind and muscles simply wouldn't move; both useless other than the bare minimum required to live and breathe. I woke up every morning that first week, my profound sadness at Mom's plight pouring from my eyes. I would sit motionless on my balcony, staring west towards the mountains of the Las Vegas valley, the only movement, raising a cup of coffee to my lips.

Mt. Charleston, or Charleston Peak, is the highest mountain in Southern Nevada, at an elevation of 12,000 feet. Its snowy peak glistened against the morning sun, even from twenty miles away. That bright sun lit reflection now a symbolic contradiction to my darkened disposition.

At this moment in time, my new business venture ceased to exist. I'd spent years planning for success and carefully calculating worse case scenarios. Where did the risks lie and how would I overcome those challenges that go with the launch of any new business? People were depending on me, and now, in the short-term, everything would be placed on hold. I never thought my mother could possibly be the reason I'd shutter my idea before it had a chance to gain traction, but I had to consider the possibility.

It required every once of mental fortitude to pretend I had a plan for Mom's future, or, now my own for that matter. I knew it would be incumbent upon me to create a workable solution for Mom, my sisters' and me.

I'd been thrust into the role of family mentor and problem solver as a young teen thanks to Dad's PTSD. In the forty years since my eighteenth birthday, my role in the family dynamic never diminished. Everyone had come to depend on me for answers. Anyone who cared to notice knew I was being slowly crushed under the weight of expectations. Within a month I quit going to the gym, and started to put on weight. I was emotionally and mentally fatigued.

I called Mom everyday just to hear her voice. I had nothing important to say. "Hi Mom, just calling to check on you." "*I'm okay, my stomach keeps bloating,*" no mention of lost memory.

I wondered how long it would be before Mom started to lose the ability to wholly care for herself? The answer to that question came just ten days after diagnosis.

She sobbed loudly, sitting in her parked car, unable to figure out which key cranked the ignition. There were only two options on Mom's key ring, one for entrée into her house, the other, a long black key from Toyota. Mom called the only number she could remember without looking in her phone book---mine. I removed the car within an hour. She would never drive again.

Karen and I merged Mom's needs into our schedules. Having my sister already living with her was a delayed blessing in disguise. My sister needed time to recover from the recession that had robbed her of a job she held over twenty years. The combination of recession and job loss eventually took my sister's home of over a decade. Mom, on the other hand needed human contact, a care monitor, and conversation with a real live voice, not some digital version emanating through a telephone.

That damn recession didn't just affect Karen; Mom lost all the equity in her home, my little sister Amanda lost her job, my son lost his job, and my investors left within six months either side of diagnosis. All of our savings were wiped out within a year. Any hope of combing financial resources to provide for Mom disappeared, we had none.

* * *

Despite the diagnosis, Mom's life went on as usual for the next two years, minus the car. The grocery store, watching football, reading books, church, the occasional walks with Rusty, complaints about her stomach, watching several hours of news, nothing truly changed. I made a decision not to share our shattered financial lives with her, she wouldn't have understood if I did.

My research into Alzheimer's intensified for a few months after diagnosis, then I fooled myself into long periods of complacency, believing Mom looked fine, when in fact, the destruction of her brain sped along quietly behind the scenes.

When I did read, it was the scientific knowledge that interested me most. It reminded me of my college days studying biology. I had an affinity for this stuff. I learned about tangles, plaques, neurons, and the hippocampus region of the brain's effect on short-term memory versus long-term, and which was likely to go first. I did extensive research into Pepto Bismal, and its affects on the brain, certain it contributed to Mom's condition.

My studies revealed that sixty to eighty percent of those with dementia had the Alzheimer's form. For those things I didn't understand, I made her doctor explain as if he were a college professor working in a lab full of student researchers.

* * *

We scheduled quarterly visits to the Cleveland Clinic for further diagnostics, treatment options, and progress monitoring.

One of the first tests required Mom to draw a clock and fill in the numbers. She passed easily. Next, the doctor asked her to draw certain times. "Anita, draw four o'clock," he said. "Now draw nine o'clock." She performed admirably given her diminished capacity, but the answers proved rather laborious, taking a full ten minutes to draw each time.

Next came questions like, what year were you born. What's today's date? How many children do you have? How many brothers and sisters do you have?

After correctly answering those questions, the doctor took out photos of three animals---an elephant, rhinoceros, and a camel. After a few moments of intense concentration, Mom couldn't identify any of them. "*I think I've seen them before.*" "Can you guess what they are," the doctor asked? A thought crossed my mind that maybe she feared providing the wrong response, worried she might get in trouble.

This would be the first time I noticed a child-like behavior in Mom that manifested itself like a fidgeting adolescent, hands and feet in constant motion, as she searched her memory for answers. I would continually be flabbergasted at the speed of diminished mental capacity. Why didn't I notice sooner? Maybe I did, but couldn't reconcile the make believe Greek tragedy that played out in my mind between Apollo and Eros--- reason versus love.

Next, the doctor verbally gave her a sequence of numbers and asked her to repeat them back---no problem. She even repeated another sequence of numbers and letters in reverse order, quickly, with little hesitation. Despite my growing fear, it had actually been a pretty good exam. The inability to remember the animals concerned me a little, but truly registered in my mind as an outlier, despite Mom's juvenile reaction when confronted with her own memory loss.

After telling the doctor I took her car, which he acknowledged was a wise move, we started talking about treatments that might, and I emphasize might, slow the progressive attack on her memory and stabilize cognitive function. We talked about Aricept, and how it, and its more generic name Donepezil, is being used to help patients.

After a lengthy discussion, the decision was made to hold off for three months. It gave me time to research the medication and how it interacted with her thyroid and blood pressure medicines.

* * *

For the next six months, Mom's mental capacity continued it's slow, nearly imperceptible decline. She'd become more sullen and withdrawn. That fierce independence still revealed itself at times, just like her mother, but the introvert, so rooted in Mom's mental makeup, marched its way to the forefront, making it easy for her to hide behind its dominance. She no longer had a desire to leave the house. Tai Chi class stopped. A few months later church stopped. When friends and family called, she refused to answer the phone. The only call she accepted was mine, only after she recognized my voice while I left a message.

She'd been on Donepezil for three months. It didn't start off so well. The drug made her drowsy. For the first time in her life, Mom walked with a cane, a prop to steady herself. At times, bright sunlight created moments of intense panic. A simple trip to the bathroom was fraught with danger. Eventually, her body adjusted and the cane went away. I didn't notice any discernable improvement in cognition, but maybe Donepezil slowed the degenerative nature of the disease. I had no way of knowing.

While I focused on the scientific facts of Alzheimer's, I completely ignored the care factor and long term needs. Another mistake I'd pay for later.

Within eighteen months of diagnosis, Mom could no longer take care of her finances. The deadly intruder continued its march through the hippocampus region of the brain on a seek and destroy mission, ruining any chance for recovery.

Her small savings account was substantially depleted, due to calculation errors and the inability to comprehend her billing statements. Bills were late, or double and triple paid. Of course no creditor would dare say she paid too much. They were happy to take the money.

Our quarterly visits to the Cleveland Clinic started to slowly reveal the progressive nature of Alzheimer's. Drawing the simple clock now proved an insurmountable obstacle. She never got the animals correct. Mom did well with her birthday, but forgot how many kids she had. She maintained her ability to manage sequences and recite numbers and letters correctly.

Mom's childish behavior led us to celebrate the smallest of achievements. I felt like placing a gold star on her paper when she got the correct answers. I held out hope things would improve, but I knew my optimism was nothing more than a temporary elixir for my tormented soul.

Karen started cooking her meals and leaving them for her to eat while she worked. Other parts of Mom's life began to crumble, except caring for Rusty. The house fell further into disrepair. Cleaning, other than washing dishes and making her bed proved impossible to consistently manage.

We now fought a battle on two fronts. The chronic stomach problems consumed more time than her memory loss. Mom could often be found doubled over in pain, rocking back and forth in a chair repositioning her body in the hope that the movement would provide relief. It was taking its toll on both her physical and mental wellbeing. Years later I discovered many Alzheimer's sufferers suffered from at least one chronic problem, but most of those were associated with the disease.

"My stomach is bloating, look at it grow, " she would cry, the loud gurgling noise audible across the room. While her stomach most definitely bloated, it certainly wasn't growing, but that was Mom's perception, which meant that was her reality.

The bloating would often be accompanied by complaints of burning and constricted throat, more than likely a symptom of acid reflux. *"I can't swallow,"* she repeated over and over again, forcing us, for a short period of time to feed her a predominantly liquid diet. Eventually we got that under control, but the gastric attacks persisted, occurring two or three times daily.

I feared at some point she would be unable to convey her symptoms to a doctor. The inability to communicate is a byproduct of late stage or severe Alzheimer's. I needed a solution to her digestive problems now. We went through three gastroenterologists, four emergency room visits, and dozens of tests over the next two years, along with visits to doctors in California---all to no avail.

No wonder Mom drank Pepto Bismal. It didn't appear any relief was on the horizon, so we attempted to manage the pain with medications prescribed by the many physicians we visited. We tried a FODMAP diet, a gluten free diet, a little exercise and more---nothing. I was so consumed with her indigestion problems, I forgot about dementia for weeks at a time, only to be reminded during our visits to the Cleveland Clinic.

By now, I hadn't worked a solid, uninterrupted week in nearly two years. From the summer of 2014 through the winter of 2015, Mom had no fewer that ten appointments a month, ninety-percent of them connected to her stomach---lab tests, MRIs, a colonoscopy, ultrasounds, CT scans---you name it we did it. The drive time alone consumed four hours daily. Her medical file was thicker than the bible on her nightstand.

During this time, Mom had quietly slipped into the moderate stage of Alzheimer's---the transition subtle and completely undetectable to us because of our laser like focus on her stomach.

* * *

Each time I took Mom to a new doctor or diagnostic lab, I would mention her Alzheimer's without explanation. As medical professionals, I just assumed they would know what that meant. Not one of them had rudimentary knowledge of the disease, often getting frustrated with Mom when she couldn't follow simple instructions, or effectively convey her thoughts and feelings. One got a little testy, forgetting his bedside manner, requiring my intervention.

I spoke with several medical professional friends, and not one had ever been trained in communicating with a person of diminished mental capacity above and beyond the obvious. Alzheimer's can be deceiving for the uninitiated, especially those in the mild or moderate stage. They look and act normal until you start a conversation.

Now when I take Mom for lab work, diagnostics, or to any doctor, I have a canned speech prepared, that often sounds threatening, although that's not my intent.

"My mother suffers from moderate stage Alzheimer's. You must repeat your instructions several times, if you want her to follow your directions. Use short declarative sentences. Please don't use compound sentences or large words. She won't remember anything you told her seconds before. I know it can be highly annoying to continually repeat yourself, but try to keep your voice neutral, Mom's very sensitive to nuance and tone. If she feels she's upset you, or you show that annoyance, she'll withdraw. If you need to make sure she's alright just ask her, 'Anita are you okay?' Anything more detailed, please make sure I'm in the room."

I altered that speech depending on the appointment or doctor, and repeat it each and every time, except at the Cleveland Clinic. As much as Mom is special to me, I no longer assume the doctors remember her. The only time I leave her side is when she changes clothes, and I demand a nurse either assist, or stand outside the door.

* * *

As a seventy-fifth birthday present, we took Mom to hear The Shirelles. Founded in 1957, the year Mom graduated from high school, this all girl group was famous, for, among other things, the hit song, *Soldier Boy.*

Mom was terrified as we entered a jam-packed indoor concert pavilion. The room easily held five hundred people, every seat occupied. She grabbed our hands holding on for dear life, one tentative step after another until we found our own seats about ten rows from the stage.

Once the music started, the gloves came off. She danced in the aisle with my girlfriend and Karen for an hour. Mom had entered a musically induced trance. I heard Alzheimer's patients respond really well to music. Well, I just witnessed that explosion of emotion and freedom first hand. Mom even remembered the lyrics and sang along like a high school kid.

* * *

Karen, unbeknownst to me at the time, started having confrontations with Mom related to the twin issues of memory loss and stomach discomfort. My sister was never one to handle stress all that well---it's not part of her mental makeup.

Mom wouldn't clean up after the dogs, even if they accidentally defecated on her bare feet. This infuriated Karen to no end, not understanding Mom's apathy was caused by dementia. Even after all my reading, I didn't get it either.

On my visits, I often found myself cleaning, unable to accept Mom living in squalor---dust on the blinds and drapes so thick you could ski on them.

Piles of dirty clothes were left unattended in the laundry room. Mom couldn't remember how to operate the washer and dryer she owned for ten years.

Mom no longer knew the difference between Clorox bleach and mouthwash. She managed to ingest some toxic chemical to brush her teeth that left her lips swollen like two inflatable rafts, her tongue the size of a small steak. We rushed to the emergency room not knowing the source of the poison. She sucked meals through a straw for a week until the swelling subsided.

The backyard looked like a minefield of dog mess, fallen leaves, leaking sprinkler valves, and dusty lawn furniture.

The home she so expertly appointed and cared for suffered from a severe case of neglect. The smell of stagnant water alerted me to one of the myriad problems left unattended until I arrived. The garbage disposal leaked water, yet Mom continued to fill it with food, grinding away it's contents. Water flooded the wooden kitchen cabinets, spilling onto the tile floor. She cleaned up the water and went back to the comfort of her chair, never once complaining about the stench.

The month before, the garage door broke. A few weeks before that, the water pipe from the sprinkler system burst during a hard freeze. A neighbor alerted Karen to the quickly freezing avalanche of water cascading down the street. The loud noise of running water splashing against the window never got Mom's attention.

Later that summer, the air conditioner unit's overflow valve leaked causing a massive whole in the garage ceiling. Mom, somehow, managed to ignore the massive whole she passed daily to empty the trash, even as a stream of water dampened her face and hair. Five thousand dollars later, Mom didn't miss a beat, leaving the backdoor open all day despite temperatures well into the triple digits.

Mom's triple digit electric bill did little to dissuade her from giving the dogs easy access to the backyard. Money and the various denominations no longer found a home in Mom's brain.

These events all occurred the year before the caregiver arrived, hence my sense of urgency to get my sister some help.

Mom confronted my sister on numerous occasions. The argument was usually over Mom's refusal to take her medications. These ultimate battle royals often required my intervention over the phone.

Then Mom took to complaining about hunger, swearing she was being starved to death despite having consumed several large meals throughout the day. Mom simply forgot she ate. The signals between brain and stomach malfunctioned.

We had no training in Alzheimer's care that could help us mitigate, what for Mom, escalated from bizarre behavior, to normal demeanor. The battles between mom and daughter intensified, typically out of my eyesight, leaving me little sympathy for my sister at the time.

When I finally confronted her, it was obvious Mom's care had pushed Karen to the brink. When I suggested looking into assisted living, she resisted, claiming she could handle things, "it's too soon for that," she would exclaim.

The next day she called, livid at something Mom had done. This back and forth went on for months. Like me, my sister was thinking with her heart, wanting the best for our mother, but unable to deliver. We finally convinced her to hire an in-home care provider, at least during work hours.

Karen immediately journeyed to Denver after the hire to watch her beloved Broncos. I stayed with Mom, cooking, cleaning and fixing things around the house. I now had a front row seat to my sister's disastrous world, and it wasn't pretty. My observations provided the impetus to move forward in pursuit of assisted living options, as long as Rusty was part of the deal.

On December 22, Mom's 76th birthday, one of the assisted living facilities held a Christmas party, in which we were all invited. Mom had the time of her life, dancing non-stop for a full thirty-minutes, resting a moment, and starting all over again. By the time we arrived home, she'd completely forgotten the experience. When I showed her the video on my cell phone, she remained in denial. The sore legs the following morning did nothing to convince her otherwise.

The Christmas party, along with the numerous dinners and movies we took Mom to, started having a positive emotional impact. She stopped complaining about her stomach and her attitude became less confrontational, almost to the point of nonexistence. My sister benefited mightily from the sudden turn of events---the kinder gentler mother appeared to be responding to these positive changes in her life. This illusion was to be short-lived.

In late January, we returned to the Lou Ruvo Brain Institute for our quarterly visit. I hit upon a thought I needed to ask the doctor about. I wanted to know if her gastrointestinal problems, and inability to detect when she was satiated could be a function of the brain and stomach sending mixed signals to each other----or no signals at all. My hypothesis was a reach, but, scientifically, at least to me, it seemed plausible, given nothing else we investigated offered a solution.

I noted over the previous months, that distracting Mom took the focus off her stomach, the pain magically disappearing, or at least subverted enough to mask its painful consequences. The doctor thought it possible, but obviously couldn't provide any conclusive evidence to support my hypothesis.

Two weeks later our worlds' came crashing down.

CHAPTER FIVE

Greed's Power

I realized we were in deep financial do-do as my father used to say when he wanted to avoid the use of expletives. I secured financial power of attorney just after Mom's diagnosis, although she maintained her own bookkeeping for another eighteen months. I quickly discovered, thanks to her poor planning and the Great Recessions, she had no assets.

The only time we ever quarreled as adults, had to do with Mom's unwillingness to make late life preparations. Death doesn't care that we argued over its inevitability, and neither did Mom. Death is there to be served, whether we accepted its finality or not.

"Mom you've got to tell me how you want to handle end of life decisions." "Mom where do you want to be buried, or would you rather be cremated?" "Mom what do you want me to do if you can no longer take care of yourself?" "Mom, have you checked your insurance policies to make sure you have enough coverage?" Those spats were exhausting.

At times she feared calling me, afraid I'd bring up the matter again. I couldn't figure out how to crack her armor, it proved impenetrable. I thought about calling her siblings, but Mom was such a private person, death wouldn't have been good enough for me in her eyes.

The canvas of our past shapes the portrait of our future. The artist, my mother, painted a nearly blank portrait that I'd now been tasked with completing, and I hated being forced to choose the colors.

As a government employee, Mom always trusted Uncle Sam would take care of her in sickness and in health. Those vows, she surmised, were stronger than marriage. I tried valiantly to share with her what I learned after my own military service, and transition to civilian life. "Mom you're going to be left high and dry," I said more times than I can count. I stressed repeatedly not to rely on government, but the crickets of silence greeted my every overture.

The time to pay the piper had arrived. Affordable care options appeared to be hopelessly nonexistent. Assisted living memory care in Nevada started at $5,500 a month, and increased exponentially depending on service needs. The basic cost alone was nearly double Mom's retirement income.

Parts of Southern California, where I hoped to return someday, had memory care facilities starting at $8,000 a month.

In-home professional care proved equally daunting for someone on fixed income with no assets to leverage. Las Vegas rates hovered between $17 and $25 per hour. At some point in the future she would require twenty-four hour care, but $400 to $600 daily was well beyond her means.

Mom's social security came with an annual cost of living increase, as did her pension. Even with that, both would lose one to three percent on an annual basis to inflation. At some point in the not to distant future, her income would not even cover basic non-memory care assisted living.

I started cutting costs immediately in a futile attempt to cover for Mom's reluctance. I paid care needs only--- mortgage, food, utilities, and anything to do with health care. I was too late.

Mom had a second problem further complicating her care needs. The recession wiped out her home equity--- the nest egg she'd come to depend on in an emergency. Despite a $58,000 down payment, back in 2006, on a $258,000 house, and making all payments on time, by early 2009, her home would be worth less than $100,000. Just reaching her loan payout left her nearly $100,000 under water, and when adjusted to the original purchase price, $158,000 below what she paid.

As of this writing, summer 2016, her home is still $40,000 under the loan balance and $120,000 less than what she paid.

If Mom's home had experienced modest equity growth of two-percent annually over ten years, it would be worth in excess of $315,000. Deducting her remaining mortgage payment, she would have had approximately $150,000 to apply to her care if she sold the home. While certainly not enough, when combined with retirement income, I could have stretched her care dollars for several years.

Taking advantage of one of the government programs enacted after the recession for people with good credit, I managed to renegotiate Mom's mortgage payment. The problem with this program, the principal remained the same. The $300 a month payment reduction was predicated on a temporary interest rate reduction. The fourth and fifth years of the renegotiated price would see those rates climb once again, meaning a higher mortgage.

So there you have it---a paltry pension losing value, social security, no savings, no home equity, and no long-term care insurance. Mom lived in a self-induced financial purgatory, exacerbated by Alzheimer's and Wall Street greed.

Basic memory care would outstrip her income by a minimum of $2,000 a month in Las Vegas. In California it would be even worse. Her income was too much to qualify for Medicaid, and even if she did, it wouldn't be enough.

Add insult to injury, she didn't qualify for any Veteran's Assistance programs, which could have provided up to $1,100 in additional income for a military spouse. My parents' were married for the entirety of Dad's military career, all twenty-one years.

They divorced a few years after his retirement. Despite the divorce, Mom would still qualify for some veteran's assistance programs, but Dad remarried about fifteen years later. The new wife is eligible for the benefits my mother earned. Dad passed away a few years back, but those benefits, as explained to me, would survive his death, if only Mom qualified. Rage doesn't adequately describe my feelings on the subject.

Mom's sacrifice would go unrewarded. Thank you for your service, now goodbye. If they only knew how much Mom loved our country and the troops she worked so hard to support. Mom was military through and through without the uniform. Now I found myself questioning whether Mom's sacrifice was worth the trouble.

Once I recognized her dilemma, I found myself wishing she'd been more selfish with her own career demands, even to the point of forcing Dad to leave military service. Seeing the world doesn't compensate for decades of low pay and lost job opportunities.

With me having poured all my assets into a new business venture, things looked bleak. Neither of my sisters' had the financial resources to help.

I investigated how others coped with Alzheimer's care financing. That investigation revealed one horror story after another of struggle and despair.

In addition to the exorbitant price of care, for those families that opted to keep their loved one at home, collectively, caregiver's lost income reached into the billions of dollars annually.

Alzheimer's and America's for profit health care system won't be sharing a seat at the dinner table anytime soon, so incompatible are the two, they make each other vomit. Sadly, there appears to be no financial solution for Alzheimer's care in the offing.

I kept thinking back to our heated arguments and realized, even if Mom had done everything right, she still wouldn't have the financial resources necessary, recession, Wall Street avarice, or otherwise.

ACT 2

"In memory everything seems to happen to music"

Tennessee Williams
The Glass Menagerie

CHAPTER SIX

First 30 Days

Week 1 --- The decision to remove Mom from her home the evening police arrived was a no-brainer. The second, more difficult decision I'd been forced to make that evening provided a moment of pause, as I processed making that removal permanent.

My sister hated us taking Mom, but realized it had to be done. She couldn't care for her no matter how badly she wanted the job.

All of mother's worldly possessions were in that home. This is it I thought to myself, a lifetime of memories, most of which Mom could no longer recollect, left behind forever.

She had artwork from our time in Spain fifty years earlier. A lifetime of family photos proudly displayed on her fireplace mantel. A closet full of clothes, many leftover from her days in the workforce, that hadn't been worn in years. Plaques and certificates of achievements adorned the walls of her home office.

Bookshelves were lined with trashy romance novels and DVDs Mom accumulated and consumed over the years. Most of this stuff was about to find itself donated or relegated to the trash heaps of history.

Why do we have so much stuff? The accumulation of things truly has no bearing on life and death. They make you happy in the moment, but at the end of the day, its nothing more than comfort food---once consumed, you either get more food, or go on a diet, a diet that in most cases fails.

The forty-five minute ride back to our apartment was quiet, save for the occasional cries coming from Rusty. He wasn't like most dogs I'd come across. He hated observing the outside world from inside a car, shaking uncontrollably at the unfamiliar surroundings and the hum of a car engine. His trepidation was probably the result of spending weeks at a time home alone with Mom. No matter how much comfort Mom provided, the nervous jitters didn't stop until we pulled into our garage.

Mom had never set foot in our new apartment of three months. With our three kids in their mid to late twenties, my girlfriend and I had no need for a large house. We traveled often, and planned to continue to do so in support of my career.

Our apartment was a new two-bedroom. We were its first tenants. It was furnished to our liking, but not one of conspicuous consumption. We both hate knick-knacks. The only items decorating our furnishings were pictures of the kids and a few plants. We were a tidy twosome. My girlfriend, and by extension me, kept our home spotless.

The second bedroom had been my home office. Now it would be converted back to its original intent.

We arrived home around 10 p.m. Mom willed her legs up the stairs, took quick inventory of her surroundings, and gingerly sat down on our new chaise lounge. None of us knew what to do, or say.

Mom looked confused, the Alzheimer's Stare on full display. That vacant look in her eyes told me she hadn't absorbed any of the night's events. I asked if she remembered the police at her house. *"No,"* she said, dumfounded.

We gave her a tour of our home. It became evident in seconds that she thought her surroundings nothing more than a hotel, and she would return to her house in a few days. Due to the lateness of the hour, we decided not to discuss the future, a prudent decision given its uncertainty.

We gathered sheets and blankets to cover our brand new sofa, Mom and Rusty's, makeshift bed until I could arrange for her bedroom furniture to be brought over. Goodnight.

My girlfriend and I hardly spoke to one another, not sure what to make of this obvious permanent disruption to our lives. My mouth was dry; palms sweaty, heart rate slightly elevated---enough to notice the pounding in my chest. We laid next to each other in bed, holding hands, staring into the darkness of the room as Mom carried on a conversation with Rusty just outside our door.

Sleep was fleeting. The clock passed 11 p.m., midnight, 1 a.m., 2 a.m. I was awake for each tick of the clock, one hour blending into the next. Time, for the moment, appeared at a standstill. I wracked my brain for solutions. None were forthcoming. I just knew my mother slept on our living room sofa, and her life now belonged to me.

I awoke early that first morning, tip-toeing into the kitchen to make a pot of coffee. Mom had already awakened, her gaze fixated on our second-story living room window, stimulated by the comings and goings of our neighbors. *"I've never seen so many people and parked cars,"* she told Rusty. *"Look pumpkin at that tall building (three stories)."*

I poured a cup of coffee and disappeared into my office, leaving her and Rusty to enjoy the view and their one-sided conversation. I sat contemplating the future, my thoughts a scattered mess. The work I intended to complete remained undone.

Unable to concentrate on work, I chose to devour the many newspapers I read online daily, as a distraction from the obvious.

My fiancé awoke around 8 a.m. and made us breakfast. Mom enjoyed the moment, seemingly happy not to be stuck in her dark dungeon of a house. The bright sunshine radiated through our large windows, its warmth adding pep to Mom's step as she gracefully glided to the kitchen table.

* * *

Mom's routine, prior to her arrival at our home was of pure monotony, better to help her manage as the world slowly disappeared. She would wake around 8 a.m. and turn on the television in her bedroom. At 8:30 a.m., Karen would give her the morning medications to be taken before breakfast. Around 10 a.m., she would leave her room fully dressed, bed made. Her first chore, open the back door for the dogs. Next, she would make herself a cup of tea and see my sister off to work.

Around 11 a.m., she would eat breakfast, usually a spinach omelet and toast. As a change of pace, she would eat a bowl of cereal with a banana.

Prior to the caregiver's arrival, it was eight hours or more of nonstop television. The only break in the action; the distractions provided by severe stomach distress. She'd watch *NCIS and Law and Order* reruns ad nauseam, followed by *Family Feud*. Mom quit watching news a year earlier, unable to keep up with the daily events of a fast-paced news cycle.

Around 2 p.m., it was lunch and another cup of tea. Lunch consisted of a bowl of soup and crackers, or a turkey sandwich. Then back to television. Neither my sister, nor the caregiver could convince Mom to take a walk in the park, she'd become so fearful of the outside world.

Despite their many attempts, Mom's steadfast refusal to budge from her sofa sent my sister into a frenzy. She complained often, a little too loudly for my taste, causing Mom to respond in kind, requiring my intervention. At other times Mom looked despondent begrudgingly accepting her sedentary lifestyle.

We didn't know enough about Alzheimer's at the time to comprehend Mom's fear, much less combat its resultant behavior. Every time I visited Mom, she would say, *"I don't get out much."* I took her words as a plea to see something beyond the four walls of her home, but the truth of the matter, Mom simply needed to hear herself speak, and for us to acknowledge she'd been heard. Her actions and words proved the ultimate contradiction.

Dinner was around 6 p.m. Before Mom lost her faculties, she'd have a meal prepared for her and Karen. Now, my sister, who doesn't cook, had a freezer loaded with easy to prepare pre-cooked meals the caregiver could just warm up. It was either pre-cooked foods, or meals ordered from a restaurant my sister would pick up on the way home.

Somewhere between 10 p.m. and 11 p.m., Mom and Rusty were back in her bedroom, television on. She'd channel surf, searching for the familiar. In the days before her memory started to disappear, she'd read for a few hours and shut everything off. Mom no longer read, preferring to watch moving images on a flat screen she couldn't comprehend.

Almost every night, as we found out later, Mom brought Rusty's food with her to bed, sprinkling his edibles across her bedspread or under the sheets. Rusty typically ignored the food. By the time I arrived to take Mom's bedroom furniture, there was enough dog food in the bedding to fill the shelves of the local grocery store.

This rather dreary life, caregiver, or no, started in earnest the year before that fateful day police were summoned. We tried in vain, to add structure and some semblance of value to Mom's daily existence, but the Devil's Disease resisted with all its might. Alzheimer's stalked its prey with reckless abandon, marching through my mother's brain on a path to destroying every relatable moment of her life.

* * *

Our first task when Mom arrived, push back on the forces of evil that had so savagely stripped her of the ability to function. We started by seeking ways to provide structure and balance. Her new surroundings demanded it, and Rusty needed it since he could no longer simply relieve himself through an open backdoor. Apartment living meant taking Rusty out for walks. A year later, Mom still opens our balcony door, thinking it's her backyard. Thankfully, Rusty got the memo.

We set breakfast for 9 a.m., lunch for 12:30 p.m. and dinner at 6 p.m., with a snack at 4 p.m. The concept of structure proved difficult for Mom to accept. It took months to regulate her eating habits. We now treat our kitchen like a restaurant, using a whiteboard to post meal times, or announce when the "kitchen is closed."

Her slow meal consumption annoys us beyond belief. I've seen a tortoise move six inches faster than it takes Mom to eat half a sandwich.

She never ate like that pre-Alzheimer's. Mom had easily become the poster child for over chewing. I read somewhere that a cow must chew its food twice to aid digestion. That's 40,000 jaw movements per day. The comparison to my mother, admittedly, is an awful one, but apt.

There were times between bites she would stare off into the abyss, trapped in the tomb of her mind, then start chewing after a long pause. I've often wondered what she might be thinking, or did she simply forget to chew.

I remember watching my grandmother eat after Alzheimer's took hold. She could be done with a four-course meal in ten minutes.

Several times throughout those early weeks, we caught Mom feeding Rusty her food from the table. No amount of screaming, hollering, admonishing, or explaining in a calm rational voice, could get Mom to quit feeding her grossly overweight dog table scraps. In fact, they weren't scraps; it was often the main course and dessert---lasagna, chicken, potatoes, yogurt, ice cream, and bread, served with a fork and spoon.

We hit on an idea that seemed to start the process of breaking the cycle. We posted a big sign on the decorative centerpiece of the table, "DO NOT FEED RUSTY." We made her read the sign at the beginning of every meal. It took a few months, but the message was delivered and received.

Sometime in Mom's past, a person of authority, or some witch doctor told her tea cured everything. The programming of Mom's subconscious to tea was something straight out of an episode of the *Twilight Zone*, or a remake of *The Manchurian Candidate*.

Mom would drink seven cups of tea, or more, daily thinking it would cure her gastrointestinal discomfort, forgetting that the previous cup did nothing, and at times made it worse.

The Devil's Disease had completely destroyed the part of the brain that allows one to process cause and effect. It would be months before we cut tea consumption down to a more healthy two cups, and get her to drink water.

Mom possessed many new idiosyncrasies and phobias that were totally unfamiliar to me. The mirage of normalcy lurked, tantalizing us with lucidity one moment, and complete irrationality the next.

Crowded places scared her; sudden movements, noise, driver's passing at normal speed all elicited some form of internal terror. Rusty being across the room and not on her lap induced panic. Fear basically controlled her every movement; real or perceived, it didn't matter. No two Alzheimer's sufferers react exactly the same to the same stimuli. None of Mom's fears and phobias would have bothered my grandmother, that 4'10" dynamo is the bravest person I knew.

* * *

My girlfriend's anxiety had reached a boiling point in just twenty-four hours. She adored Mom, and the feeling was mutual, but that "not again look on her face," told me all I needed to know.

Mom's paranoid repetitive behavior wore on both of us, only I couldn't act on my angst. My lady and I talked constantly that first day, and every day thereafter for weeks, usually at my insistence. It seemed to help both of us, but I knew we couldn't continue with our ad hoc counseling sessions. We would need to speak with someone outside the house who had more experience with this disease.

Mom would have been crushed at the thought of me losing someone over her. It took several months for us to find a balance, and even then, I am very much aware it's an uneasy truce that could blow up in our face at any moment. The doctor's admonition three years earlier to seek a support group had finally found a home in my conscious.

My girlfriend expressed her own frustration by talking to her own mother, the day after Mom arrived. She needed an outlet other than me; one I felt duty bound to support. I never asked about the tenor of those conversations believing it a private matter. She did say her mother encouraged my sweetheart to stay and help, but I didn't push for more information.

I was reminded we were racing against a rapidly moving clock, not one whose speed could be measured by earth's orbit around the sun, but more by a bullet fired from an AK-47. The synapses of Mom's brain were rapidly losing the battle over control of her mind, and would eventually lead to loss of control over certain bodily functions.

I dread the thought of what the future might hold if she were left in my incapable hands.

By now, in my unscientific analysis, Mom progressed to a midway point of the moderate stage. The next stop would be the devil's total control of Mom's body, occasionally allowing us a glimpse of the real woman I loved so dearly.

* * *

On day three, we started getting Mom out of the house. First, we took Rusty to the groomer. Mom panicked at the thought of leaving him. By the time they'd both come to live with us, Rusty hadn't been groomed in a year, his nails so long they curled under his paws, causing considerable pain.

The trip to the groomer proved beyond any reasonable doubt I could no longer treat Mom like my mother, but more as a dependent toddler with adult tendencies. I bribed her with a snack so she would relinquish control of Rusty. Distraction and bribery, if necessary, would become part of my Alzheimer's arsenal. It helped me create the illusion that she was in control, when if fact, she was not.

Every lesson we taught her from this point forward required constant reinforcement with no guarantees. I became intimately familiar with the word patience, something that doesn't come easy to me.

My girlfriend's stress levels continued to rise despite our communications and positive encouragement from her family. I found myself soothing her emotions and Mom's one right after the other, leaving me no room to work out my own frustration. My girlfriend kept assuring me she was in this for the long haul, but I was doubtful. Too much happened too fast to allow me any comfort.

I needed her help, but I didn't want my desperation to be the reason she stayed. I hadn't depended on anyone since childhood. Now I had to look myself in the mirror and admit I couldn't do this alone. While her and Mom had a bond, it wasn't a fifty-eight-year legacy. That freed her to convince me to make some tough decisions for the better, that I might not have considered vital, such as simply putting Mom on a schedule and enforcing the rules, rules that quite frankly Mom doesn't remember.

* * *

Mom took to our excursions away from the house like fire to dry kindling wood, once we managed her mistrust of public spaces. The warming springtime temperatures certainly seemed to help. She commented often about the warmth, like she discovered sunlight for the first time.

We took her to breakfast the same morning Rusty went to the groomer. A day later, it was the grocery store, followed by a manicure and pedicure. Her hands and feet looked terrible, frightening the poor woman charged with providing the service.

When the technician told Mom to put her feet in the water, you'd have thought we asked her to disrobe in public until she looked around at the other customers. Once the warm water gushed over those parched feet, she relaxed.

The technician worked feverishly, scraping away dead skin, leaving the surrounding floor looking like a recent snowstorm struck the area. Her toenails curled back under her feet like Rusty's paws.

Her fingernails were equally disgusting and could easily be classified a health hazard. Mom never allowed herself to enjoy the spoils of life, even a simple mani/pedi. She handled all of her personal hygiene, leaving only her hair to be done by a professional. Anything short of perfection would not stand. Dementia stole that part of her identity.

The first time she ever allowed anyone to do her nails, was the year prior, when I took her for the first time. I didn't know what to ask for, trusting the people to point me in the right direction. Now I'm an expert on fills, paraffin wax, tips and coloring.

When the manicurist asked Mom to pick a color for her nails, she hesitated, before I realized, she couldn't name the colors. Orange, red, purple---those names meant nothing, and she didn't think to simply point.

I took a photo of her pampering with my cell phone and looked back at it later. The Alzheimer's Stare so deep and prevalent in her eyes. Any new experience from this point forward had a shelf life of recognition and enjoyment that lasted no more than a nanosecond.

A week later she complained so much about the nail polish, and how it came to be applied, we were forced to remove it. Mom wasn't upset about the color as far as I could tell; it was polish in general.

* * *

We managed to convince Mom to sit on our balcony, after a week of combating another one of her fears, the fear of heights, a hang-up that preceded Alzheimer's. I knew she would enjoy the experience. As a family, we would congregate on the front porch of my grandparents' home in Atlantic City after dinner. We would laugh, joke, or simply dose off as blood rushed to our stomachs digesting another of my grandmother's sumptuous meals. It was a memory from the distant past I'm certain she retained, her memory of Atlantic City so strong.

Eventually, we placed a radio on the balcony to entice her to stay. She would watch the planes from a distance and tell Rusty of her excitement. *"See pumpkin"* one of her nicknames for Rusty, *"the planes are going really fast." "Oh, pumpkin there goes another* one. *It's a different color."* *"See pumpkin, the wheels (landing gear) are coming out."* *"Did you see that pumpkin?"* Rusty contorted his little body trying to make sense of it all.

At times, she would talk to Rusty asking questions and await a verbal response. If I didn't know better, it would have been a cute exchange, like that between a little girl and her doll. Then, as if to make an excuse for his lack of response, Mom would tell Rusty, *"If you don't want to talk to me, that's ok."* We never interrupted those moments. It just didn't seem appropriate.

* * *

Every Sunday for the past two years, my girlfriend and I ate Sunday brunch with her parents'. My future mother-in-law would start preparing the day before. They lived in one of Las Vegas's top retirement communities' minutes from our apartment. We thought about taking Mom, but decided she'd been through enough this first week. Introducing her to new people so soon, seemed, at the time, like a bad idea.

I thought about my own grandparents' when I look at my girlfriend's parents'. My grandparents' embraced all life had to offer---they lived life, life didn't live them. When they passed away, both at age ninety-five, as much as I hated to lose them, we knew they'd squeezed every once of enjoyment out of living; nothing was left undone.

Mom, on the other hand, had become a hermit in recent years. Given she had lived alone for small stretches of time the past year, we thought, we could leave her for two hours. This proved to be another miscalculation on my part that bordered on insanity, mine.

When we returned, Mom was warming a lasagna TV dinner on the hotplate of our coffee pot. Chemicals from under the kitchen sink sat on the counter next to the food she tried to warm. Uncertain whether she mixed the chemicals with the food, we threw everything in the trash infuriating her to no end. We quickly provided her with our leftovers and Mom's anger subsided.

My inability to fully accept Mom's mental decline could have caused her considerable harm, up to and including death. How many more near mishaps did I have to experience before I woke the hell up?

Well, we acted by purchasing childproof locks for the kitchen. We banned her, politely of course, from the kitchen, including tea making. We prepared all her meals. I knew she wouldn't mind, Mom hated cooking even on her best days of life.

The first time Mom heard the microwave emit its humming sound, she screamed frantically, sprinting back to the comfort and safety of her room. When the buzzer alerting us the food was ready beeped, she acted as if we needed to evacuate.

Mom would never be left alone again.

* * *

Many Alzheimer's patients are wanderers, known to leave the comfort of their homes with no particular destination in mind. That isn't the case with our Mom, her innate fear of the unknown washes over her in a tidal wave of panic.

We've never worried she would leave the house. Besides, we had a built-in home deterrent. Our apartment required climbing stairs to reach the living level, and Mom feared stairs more than strange places. We contemplated placing a gate to cover the stairway entry, but thought it better to leave it open, using fear to our advantage.

Instead of wandering, Mom paces back and forth like a caged lion, making frequent trips between her bedroom and the balcony. The constant to and fro created a slight crevasse in our faux hardwood floors. She could make a dozen trips an hour, not remembering any of the previous journeys.

When a delivery truck comes to a neighbor's house, or the trash truck spins around the corner, Mom's eyes widened in terror *"They're not coming up here are they?"* We often found Mom trembling in her room until the offending truck fled the scene.

During the evening hours, Mom would make her way to each and every room in the house like she'd been ordered to participate in some clandestine military operation. She closed all the blinds, fearful neighbors were watching from across the street.

"I don't want people looking into my house" she'd exclaim in a belligerent and defiant tone. *"They can see right into my bedroom."* Before I learned how to handle Alzheimer's patients, and their often-false assumptions, I challenged her observations, directly, with no reservations about the harm it might cause. That approach typically brought a hostile rebuke.

* * *

The following morning, I made a trip to Mom's home to gather more of her belongings---photos, her bible, clothes, and small mementos.

We decided to simplify her life in response to information Karen provided. Mom would remove half the clothes from her spacious walk-in closet, trying to decide what to wear for a journey from the bedroom to the kitchen. The search could easily last an hour.

In a week, I no longer recognized my own mother. Who was this woman? Who was this stranger in our midst? This beautiful woman's brain had been under assault for at least three years, probably longer. Some aspects of her personality remained intact, those introverted ways being chief among them. On the other hand fears, phobias, occasional hallucinations, and behavioral distortion, claimed significant portions of her new personality.

Except Mom's fear of the outside world, which had lessened somewhat since her arrival, none of the other personality changes had a discernable pattern.

Sadly, the elevator started to descend, picking up speed gradually, now perceptible to the human eye. The emergency brakes would never engage to save her from the unrelenting ravages of this disease. The best I could hope for was to slow the elevator down.

Medical breakthroughs were years away, and even if they found a cure tomorrow, it would be too late. The only question that remained, how much time did she have before the elevator crash-landed, a question I asked her doctor a few years earlier---five years, ten, fifteen, we were still no closer to an answer. Outward appearances told me we were looking at a minimum ten years.

CHAPTER SEVEN

Search for Relief

Week 2 --- I heard the phrase "take care of yourself," no fewer than a dozen times the year before Mom's arrival. When I first received that counsel, I admittedly didn't understand the inference. The pressure put on caregivers by an Alzheimer's sufferer, family, or not, is tremendous. The burden and responsibility that goes with providing care is suffocating to the uninitiated. It could easily lead to bouts of depression or worse if you're not careful.

After one week, I needed advice and a dose of levity. Studying the effects of this disease, and actively participating in the laboratory experiment that is my mother, left me feeling, at times, like a violent earthquake caved in the walls of my home, trapping me under heavy rubble.

My aunt and I spent forty-five minutes on the phone one afternoon. What she said about my grandparents', their suffering and hers, was frightening, yet she managed to lace our chilling conversation with humor only she could provide.

Back and forth we went on an emotional roller-coaster, serious one-minute, uncontrollable laughter the next. She inquired about my wellbeing. "How are you holding up? I feigned ignorance to the true meaning of her question, a Herculean effort given Mom's Alzheimer's had already beaten me into a mild depressive state. I remain uncertain if she detected the distress in my voice.

In a moment of immense humility for my dear aunt, she admitted being on the verge of an epic meltdown before family intervened, giving her a well-earned vacation. Unless I could come up with some financial windfall, the best I could hope for were a few stolen hours of occasional relief. The enormity of what lay in front of me, if I didn't understand before this conversation, was driven home with a painful clarity that hence forth, I would have to embrace to survive.

My aunt deftly switched the conversation to a pleasant memory we both shared. She teased me, with great joy, about my toddler years and the song I used to sing, *Walk Like a Man*, by The Four Seasons. I would walk around my grandparents' house singing that tune nonstop for hours at a time. Her imitation of my little three or four-year-old self had me in stitches. The levity proved a good elixir for the moment.

* * *

We started our search for in-home care at the local Alzheimer's Association. I sought, at a minimum, twice-weekly relief from mommy care. Between phone calls and emails, we were flooded with alternatives within a week. We sifted through pamphlets in search of answers, affordable, or otherwise.

While waiting for other care information to arrive, I called Medicare, her primary health insurance provider, and Aetna her secondary insurer. They had nothing to supplement care costs. I knew that before I called, but I needed to hear it from them, on the off chance a program might exist I hadn't heard of previously.

Next came the Social Security Administration. I expected and received the same answers as those from her health insurers---nothing. She'd been receiving social security since retirement ten years earlier, but again, I needed confirmation.

Then, came the call to a veteran's support organization, that due to some arcane rules, were unable to recognize Mom's sacrifice and contribution to Dad's career.

Despite their kindness, this rebuke for assistance stung more than any other. Her love of the military and her sacrifice would not be reciprocated. At the time of my parents' divorce, Mom was entitled to half Dad's retirement income. The kind soul that Mom is, she refused, despite every important person in her life, me included, urging her to take the money. Instead, she took just $200 a month, plus child support for my younger sister. Since Dad passed three years ago, even that $200 was now gone.

After hanging up the phone, I cursed more than I had in years, and that's saying a lot. Nobody, except my girlfriend and my son escaped my wrath. "F" bombs flew from my mouth in a fit of rage I hadn't exhibited my entire life.

"How in the "f***ing hell could they not have a contingency in place for situations like Mom's," I yelled, pounding on the kitchen counter. My girlfriend just stood in silence, unable to respond. "Certainly, there were other divorcees of military retirees that needed assistance," I said, slowly calming myself.

It took thirty minutes before I regained control of my emotions and made my next call to the Department of Health and Human Services, Aging & Disability Services Division, State of Nevada. It would be two weeks before a counselor returned my call.

Once again I would be disappointed. Mom's income exceeded the maximum income threshold by nearly $1,500. To qualify for any benefits, her maximum income would need to be no more than $2,194, with less than $2,000 in assets. Even at those levels, assisted care had to be partially paid for by the recipient.

I mentioned how ridiculous those figures sounded. "This is Nevada," I bellowed, my blood pressure spiraling northward. If I couldn't get a grip on my mounting displeasure with the system, it would be me in need of medical care. "The minimum cost of memory care in Las Vegas is $5,500 a month," I shouted, "significantly more, by the time these facilities started nickel and diming people to cover the extra resources necessary to provide appropriate levels of care for an Alzheimer's patient." The counselor remained silent as I ranted, obviously well trained in the art of ignoring ill-mannered people such as myself.

"How much do you supplement Medicaid recipients' income," I screamed. "You obviously don't pay $2,000 a month in additional support," which would leave an Alzheimer's patient well short of the minimum required for care. I didn't listen for an answer, by now seething at the ridiculousness of the process. I'd stopped thinking about my mother. My argument now centered on the lack of stronger support throughout the entire system.

Long-term care insurance was out of the question. Mom needed coverage now, and long-term care insurance was a phenomenon of the last twenty years.

Next, I turned to the possibility of a reverse mortgage so prominently marketed to senior citizens on television. I quickly dismissed that idea, knowing Mom's home was still underwater thanks to the rapaciousness of Wall Street.

One solution, presented to me by the Alzheimer's Association is a $500 voucher to pay for care at an approved facility, or, in-home by an approved care provider. Once those funds are exhausted, you can apply for a supplemental for an additional $500, if there are any remaining funds. These vouchers are good once per fiscal year.

I would find another voucher a few months later through Helping Hands of Vegas Valley that paid $1,000 annually.

These vouchers are marketed as a respite service for the care provider. The funds do nothing to address the financial burdens of long-term care, but after our early experiences with an Alzheimer's patient, we were overjoyed at the prospect of taking a short break to recharge our batteries.

Dementia research and care is the least funded of all the major diseases, not just in the United States, but globally. America itself is at the nucleus of an Alzheimer's tsunami, the massive wave rushing toward humanity at breathtaking speed. It has the potential to crush families and our for-profit health care system. A story I recently watched on the CBS News program *60 Minutes*, suggests there are 1,000 new cases of Alzheimer's diagnosed in the United States daily.

Why isn't more being done? Our increasing life spans dictate an increase in the number of cases. That 5.4 million diagnosed with Alzheimer's in America in 2016, seemed a little short of a realistic number, given the recent change in reporting standards. Experts predict Alzheimer's sufferers in the U.S. will reach nearly 14 million by 2050.

That same afternoon as I made these calls, my girlfriend visited the local grocery store, where she overheard a cashier's conversation with a customer about her mother-in-law's bout with Alzheimer's and their struggles. The ugly reality had been put on full display for all in earshot. You could feel the angst and frustration in her voice, I was told. Incidents like this would continue for weeks, as if the universe were moving Alzheimer's into our orbit, providing information, and letting us know we were not alone.

* * *

Caring for Mom is tantamount to a major science experiment. I continually posit a hypothesis, and test the various solutions in the laboratory, better known as our house.

One of those tests involves time. I needed to occupy Mom's waking hours. Sitting around watching television twelve hours a day, like she'd done the previous few years is totally unacceptable, at least to me. It seems like a huge waste of time, especially when one considers Mom's limited comprehension.

The first afternoon of her second week, we purchased a small card table for her room, and a three hundred piece puzzle. Mom loved puzzles. During my youth, we often built two and three thousand piece behemoths on our kitchen table, forcing the family to eat on TV trays for weeks at a time.

After I left home, Mom continued her fascination with puzzles, often framing the finished product for use as home decorations.

I hoped the sight of a puzzle would trigger some distant pleasurable memory. The side benefit, of course, forcing her mind to work in an attempt to stall declining cognition. I worried three hundred pieces might be too much, but it mattered little at the moment. Our first experiment had begun.

Mom struggled the first few days building the border. We intervened by separating out the flat-edged pieces. It took her a week to complete that border. She was so proud of her accomplishment she bolted from her room imploring us to come see. We didn't want to let the moment pass, so we rewarded her with an ice cream sandwich. This felt so juvenile for a woman of Mom's stature, but we didn't know what else to do, so we enjoyed the ride.

Next, we divided the puzzle into sections. We thought it better to simplify the process. As days went by, Mom's concentration diminished. She focused in thirty-minute intervals, then twenty, then fifteen. Then she would go days without touching the puzzle. Had our experiment failed, or did she simply need more variety? At the moment, I didn't have an answer. I would later determine that solitary endeavors had limited reward.

* * *

The new meal structure started to take hold, when moments before our 10 p.m. bedtime, I heard rustling in the kitchen. I arrived to see Mom fighting with the refrigerator door, in a violent struggle for supremacy. She pulled with all her might, but those darn childproof locked doors wouldn't budge. "Do you need something Mom," I asked in a calm voice. I'd already looked into her eyes and noted the Alzheimer's Stare. No sense getting upset, it would only lead to further confusion.

"*I need to eat something*," she exclaimed in a slightly agitated voice. "*I haven't eaten all day, and I want some ice cream.*" I made a huge mistake, a mistake another aunt would warn me about a few months later, "DON'T EXPLAIN."

"Mom, you had three meals, a snack, and cheesecake after dinner." She slammed her fist on the kitchen counter screaming, "*you're a liar*" in a deep guttural tone, that sounded like it came up from the depths of hell. The rage coursed through every fiber of her being. Her inflection reminiscent of a scene out of a horror movie, aided by special sound effects meant to illicit just the right level of fright to scare the hell out of the viewer.

Well, it worked, except, my reaction wasn't one of jitters, I became enraged, about to pounce like a coiled snake ready to inject a painful venomous bite. My girlfriend intervened, pulling me towards our bedroom. I needed to disengage from the impending battle.

I could hear their conversation, ease dropping through the partially cracked door. "*I don't remember eating all that food, no I didn't*" Mom yelled, voice still dripping with rage. My girlfriend stood her ground. It took Mom five minutes to gather herself, but I could tell she'd gotten under my girlfriend's skin.

I regained my composure, walked into the kitchen, and looked Mom directly in her eyes. She'd completely forgotten her explosion. She shot me one of those loving looks only mothers can give. I didn't know what to make of the sudden change in demeanor, but decided to go with it, choosing to deescalate rather than create a winners and losers scenario.

My lady, in another stroke of genius, told Mom we would create a daily food log to help her memory. *"I just don't remember,"* punishing herself for a lapse in memory she was only beginning to realize she had no control over. In a matter of moments, Mom had transformed from extreme agitation to tears. I reached up and gave her a hug, despite my residual indignation at what had just transpired.

The idea of a daily food log resonated with Mom. Years earlier, I created one on a calendar to help her with weight loss, per her doctor's request, and to discover what might be causing severe gastrointestinal distress. Mom filled in that chart religiously. While we never solved her stomach problems, she did lose weight.

By 10:30 p.m., we were all in bed exhausted from the first of a series of heated exchanges over the next few months, usually all about her stomach and that damn bloating.

* * *

I awoke at 4 a.m., after another restless night of sleep. I drank coffee on the darkened balcony refusing to turn on a single light. Ninety minutes later I was greeted with a gorgeous burnt orange sunrise. Birds chirped some delightful tune happy to see another day. I watched as they scurried about from one rooftop to the next, without a care in the world. If only I had their life.

I thought about all the friends and colleagues who commended me for taking care of Mom. "I'm so proud of you big guy." Why, at this moment, didn't I feel the same way?

I couldn't bring myself to see the positive after Mom's explosion. I took her calling me a liar personally. I knew it was the Devil's Disease, but at the moment the fresh sting still bled a little, and kept me from accepting that truth.

* * *

My girlfriend needed to run a few errands. While away, I took it upon myself to have Mom take a shower. I should have waited, but wanted to prove to myself, I could handle her minimum care needs. Besides, Mom still bathed herself I just needed to provide a prompt.

Mom happily complied, but had a few questions of her own. *"How do I turn on the shower?" "Where is the soap?" "Where is the towel and washcloth?"* Had I bitten off more than I could chew?

I turned on the water making sure it wasn't too hot, just like I did for my son when he was younger. She repeatedly asked about the soap, towel, and washcloth as gallons of precious water swirled down the drain, steam obscuring the view from the bathroom mirror.

Finally satisfied with all my answers, I stepped out to give her privacy. I placed a chair outside the door and sat drinking coffee. Rusty took up position underneath the chair. We both sat, like expectant fathers-to-be in a hospital waiting room. My mind started racing for the umpteenth time since her arrival. Would she fall and bang her head? Would she know how to turn the water off? Would she actually use the soap I put on the washcloth, or simply ignore it, like most little kids left to their own devices?

Dozens of questions ran through my mind as the water continued to run. It occurred to me while she showered, there were no clean clothes in the bathroom. I quickly gathered underwear, bra, pants and shirt, slipped into the bathroom undetected and removed the dirty clothing, replacing it with clean attire.

The thought of possibly seeing Mom naked made me cringe. It felt so inappropriate regardless of circumstances, short of life and death. Whew, catastrophe averted.

I reclaimed my mantle outside the bathroom door and waited. The shower went off, then silence. "Are you okay," I shouted through the door. *"I'm okay."* Rusty looked at me satisfied his mommy would survive and returned to what had become his chair in Mom's bedroom. Note to self: don't have Mom take a shower without a female present.

Mom asked me for her third cup of tea that morning, which I declined, convincing her water was a healthier option. She accepted my explanation without comment and returned to the balcony to watch airplanes.

When my girlfriend returned, I told her the joyous news of how I got Mom to shower, proud of myself for having accomplished such an arduous task. She looked at me, laughed, and gave Mom some body lotion to apply to her extremely dry arms and feet. I guess I hadn't truly completed the mission at hand.

*   *   *

I restarted Mom on Donepezil. A drug prescribed by the Lou Ruvo Brain Institute to help with cognition. She'd been off the drug for two weeks. Since I wasn't around on a daily basis the previous year, I had no idea if it helped. I took copious notes over the next few weeks. "Mom acted a little lethargic today." "Mom seemed tired." "Mom didn't remember eating her meal just five minutes ago." "Mom talked to Rusty like a human and got mad at him for not answering her." "I asked Mom about her puzzle, while standing next to her puzzle table, her response, what puzzle."

I called my aunt and inquired about the drug. My grandmother also took Donepezil. When her doctor failed to recognize any improvement, she was taken off the medication. Only time would tell if my mom met the same fate.

*   *   *

After two hours of sleep, I awoke once again before sunrise. I sat at my desk for no more than a minute when

I heard the faint noise of crumpled paper coming from Mom's room. What was she doing awake before dawn. I crept to the door, opened it ever so slightly, so as not to create a disturbance. She was reading one of the two bibles she owned under a dim lamplight.

I watched unnoticed. I could see her mouth the words, lips moving slow and deliberate. I didn't care if she understood a single word; bless her heart, she was trying. The gratified look on her face brought a smile to mine. I closed the door as softly as I had opened it and went back to work.

When I entered her room again at 8 a.m. to take Rusty for a walk, she was in REM sleep, eyeballs fluttering violently beneath closed lids. Something played out beneath those eyelids; I just wish I knew if it was a pleasant experience for her. Rusty's violent movement as he leapt off the bed did nothing to upset the cadence of her breathing.

Fifteen minutes later the dream ended, with Mom acting as if she just ran a 10K, breathing heavily. That's how she slept I discovered, in thirty-minute intervals, followed by several hours of leisure activity, then back to sleep for another thirty-minutes, 24/7. Her lack of consistent, uninterrupted sleep, I knew, was dementia related.

Later that day, we ordered Chinese food and watched the Academy Award winning film *Spotlight* on pay per view. Mom sat quietly, her eyes following the action on television. She struggled with comprehension, drawing a complete blank when I asked her how she enjoyed the film so far.

Unwilling and/or afraid to interrupt our enjoyment, she simply sat, staring into space, no longer focused on television, rather my girlfriend's son, someone she hadn't met before. Mom retreated to the safety of her room, backing through the door with a wary eye towards the stranger in her midst.

I followed more out of curiosity. Alone, she asked about the gentleman sitting in our living room. Numerous explanations did little to eliminate the confusion, but she seemed satisfied we were safe and had me turn on her television. I tried shows I thought she might recognize from back in the day, *The Jeffersons*, *Murder She Wrote*, *Gunsmoke*, and reruns of *I Love Lucy*. None of it hit home. It was *Wheel of Fortune*, *Family Feud* or bust---Channel 1344 on Cox cable. The Game Show Network would become her video companion of choice.

* * *

I had two deadlines rapidly approaching now complicated by Mom's arrival. In forty-five days we were scheduled to leave the country on a seven-day business trip. After days of careful self-deliberation, I called Amanda in California in search of a sitter, willing to come to our house. She agreed. Despite my overture, I had serious reservations.

California sister had only seen Mom once in six years. Mom had no memory of her. In fact, Mom had no recollection of her other daughter, the one she lived with the previous three years.

I started preparing Mom for her daughter's arrival by scheduling weekly Skype calls. Mom didn't know what to make of Skype, pushing the laptop away. She thought seeing her daughter on a computer screen was some kind of hocus-pocus. Mom eventually accepted the advance in technology, but remained cautious---strange behavior coming from a former computer technician.

Amanda didn't truly know what she signed up for. The Mom she remembered on her previous journey last year, mentally, was lost to the ages. Like me, there would be painful lessons ahead.

California sis and I spoke several times a week. I explained everything I could think of---fear, hallucinations, paranoia, short-term versus long-term memory loss, and how all of it applied to Mom in its various forms. "Use short, simple sentences to communicate," I said. "Tell her what you want, and repeat it several times if necessary. If she gets upset or frustrated about something that doesn't involve endangering herself, or others, quickly change the subject."

When Mom's stomach starts to bloat, she feels more food is necessary despite having eaten a generous meal ten minutes earlier. "Give her a Lifesaver candy," I said, "she believes they are antacids pills. Usually the bloating, real or perceived, passes in thirty minutes."

My little sister fears nothing, its just not part of her DNA. She is one tough cookie. She would need to rely on that internal strength to get through her week on the battlefield of Mom's mind.

The second deadline worried me more. My girlfriend would be gone for a month, leaving me to handle Mom alone, while she tended to the birth of her first granddaughter. Outwardly, I was a cool customer, but inside, I was terrified. My mind flooded with the waters of failure, not success. I'd already decided not to work that month, falling further and further behind all my career aspirations, but I didn't have much of a choice at the moment.

* * *

I stopped by Mom's house once again, this time to gather important papers. I found her high school diploma, class of 1957, Atlantic City High School. Next, I discovered my own birth certificate and another certificate of live birth issued by the hospital. I'd never seen that certificate of live birth. I studied the little baby feet ink pattern smeared on the respective squares of the document. I couldn't help but smile at my discovery, given I'm now 6'4" and wear a size 15 shoe.

I located our single passport from 1962, when we journeyed to Spain, as part of Dad's military career. Plastered on the passport was the stamp of entry into Madrid, and photos of Mom, the older of my two little sisters', and me. California sis would be conceived in

Spain, and born shortly after our return to the United States three years later.

I rushed home, excited to share my discovery. I'm certain Mom hadn't seen these documents in years. I showed her the diploma first, and the program from her graduation ceremony with classmates names. None of it registered except the name Atlantic City.

I showed her the certificate of my live birth. A smiled pursed her lips at the site of two inkblots representing my baby feet. Finally a connection, I thought. I asked if she knew whose certificate she held. *"That's my son."* "Anita, that's Michael," my girlfriend said, pointing at me, a sharp finger jab to my chest. *"That's you,"* she inquired, *"That's so cute."* Okay, moving on.

I handed her the passport. She looked, and didn't quite recognize herself for a moment. The she looked at me; *"When did I take this?"* Without answering I asked, "Do you remember going to Spain? We lived there for three years." *"I know we went across the ocean,"* she proudly proclaimed. She always remembered the ocean, her first plane ride, ecstatic she'd survived what she thought was a treacherous journey.

Then she wanted to know about the three and five-year-old, whose photos adorned her passport. "Anita, that's Michael, that's him," my girlfriend said, once again pointing, in a decidedly louder voice than the previous reference. I immediately shutdown the conversation, fearful Mom would get upset at her inability to recall.

* * *

At 3:45 a.m. we hear a muffled noise coming from the kitchen. It's Mom, fully dressed. I enter the room, look directly into her eyes and know immediately she's confused---the "Alzheimer's Process Look." It's different than the "Alzheimer's Stare." The "Process Look" is one of attempted recognition. The countenance between the two is decidedly different.

She looked back and forth, placing furniture. She surveyed the kitchen, but couldn't quite place all the appliances and kitchen cabinetry. The cabinets in her home were a light pinewood; ours a shaker style with a dark cherry wood stain.

Then she glanced at the stairs leading down to the garage. After another moment of silence, she spotted what she thought looked familiar; a door leading to what she believed was her backyard.

She looks at Rusty, and leads him to the balcony thinking he would relieve himself. The balcony and the darkness at that hour proved a little disorienting. Mom beat a hasty retreat from the night sky. "Mom, it's the middle of the night, it's supposed to be dark outside." She gave me that "Are you sure?" look.

Time references mean nothing to Mom. To Mom, day is night and night is day, it's all the same. Noon could just as easily be midnight.

Once she got her bearings, Mom reopened the door and commenced pushing and prodding poor Rusty to relieve himself on the balcony. *"Well, if you don't hurry up, I'm going back inside.*" Rusty knew the balcony wasn't the place and beat a hasty retreat of his own to the stairs leading outdoors. Mom looked puzzled.

My girlfriend finally spoke up. "Anita, you are not at your home, you are in our house, Michael's and mine." *"No, this is my house, I've been living here for ten years,"* Mom shouted in defiance. For the next twenty minutes, we talked to Mom about where she now lived. Nothing made sense as Rusty paced, desperate to empty his little bladder.

After a moment of contemplation, Mom said, *"I woke up because Rusty told me he had to go to the bathroom."* "How did he tell you," my girlfriend asked? *"He looked at me and told me he had to go."* I was halfway down the stairs when she made that comment.

Rusty was out and back in less than a minute. He drank a little water then gave Mom the "time to go back to bed look." Rusty's internal body clock proved too hard for Mom to resist. *"Let's go back to bed pumpkin."* With that, they returned to her bedroom. I turned on her television and told her I'd be back in a few hours for breakfast.

I entered her bedroom at 9 a.m. to give her a cup of tea, like I'd done every morning the previous two weeks. Her light snoring flashed like a do not disturb sign. I retreated leaving her to catch up on some much needed rest.

* * *

It's the second day in a row Mom had awakened before the sun appeared on the eastern horizon. Bleary-eyed, I drank two cups of coffee in fifteen minutes, praying for an adrenalin rush. I'd always enjoyed the peace and solitude of early mornings, now I felt violated.

Rather than rest, or catch up on my reading, I'd started to master the art of cramming a days worth of work into a three-hour window. I still had no idea how I was going to run a new business that would arguably require me to work fifteen hours a day, but I had to try. I'd invested too much to turn back now. Things that required my utmost concentration had to be accomplished before sunrise, or before mom-rise, otherwise, it might never get done.

The lack of sleep two mornings in a row left me feeling a tad cranky, ready to explode at the slightest provocation. Ninety minutes after I sat down to work, Mom emerged ready to take on the day's challenges. That was all the provocation I needed, practically throwing my computer through the window, before I restrained myself, just as it was about to leave my hands.

For the next two hours I entertained Mom, talked to her, tolerated her constant pacing from the bedroom to the balcony and back, her incessant whining about her stomach, followed by, *"Has Rusty eaten yet?"* "He will eat at 9 o'clock when I feed you," I repeated a half-dozen times before I changed the subject, only to have her broach it once again minutes later.

Mom exhibited this excessive/compulsive behavior many times throughout the day, primarily on matters of Rusty's wellbeing.

I made her a cup of hot tea, the aphrodisiac of beverages, as far as Mom is concerned. Tea and ice cream were her comfort foods---give her either one, she'd be quiet for an hour. I used the diversion to rush through some mindless parts of my work. An hour later, that cup of tea was untouched, yet she held that porcelain container in a vice-like grip, daring anyone to pry it from her hands.

That was our day from dawn until dusk and beyond. Between her incoherent thoughts, constant pacing, hysterical outbursts, and our need to make sure she didn't injure herself, Mom managed to consume two adults on a fulltime basis.

I needed a support system, but hadn't had time to cobble one together other than my aunt. This was the one time in my life where being cool under pressure worked to my detriment. Every positive emotion I could muster now under full assault.

I started talking to anyone who would listen---friends, other family members, and business partners. I needed them in ways I couldn't effectively communicate. Once again, everyone told me how proud they were I'd taken on mommy care. I just wasn't there yet, too tired, and upset to accept the obvious complement.

One of my new business partners lived through what we now experienced. While no two dementia sufferers manifest their behavior in exactly the same manner, the pressure and strain placed upon the caregiver/s had similarities that couldn't be denied.

We talked for an hour after a meeting, me desperately seeking wisdom and relief. He asked me what kind of personality Mom had pre-Alzheimer's. I thought to myself, what a strange question, but answered, knowing he was going somewhere with his thoughts. "She was the ultimate introvert," I responded. "She could sit in a room with one other person, and that other person wouldn't know she was breathing."

"Introverts keep feelings bottled up inside, but at times can express themselves in fits of anger, that might come as a complete surprise," he said. "The memory that provided a filter on your mother's true feelings died with the disease." It proved to be a very prescient observation on his part, and conveyed to me like the lawyer he was---logical and straight to the point. I just listened, unable to refute or verify its veracity.

* * *

We installed a phone in Mom's bedroom. She never called anyone except me, but her family and best friend called often. I hoped she would answer and engage in conversation. It wasn't long before I discovered that phone was like an uninvited guest, its ring preying upon her psyche to devastating consequences. Mom's friend, sisters', brother, and her daughter called in about a five-hour time span after the phone went live. Each time the phone rang, Mom became panic-stricken, running from her room on occasion at warp speed, breathing heavily; *"Michael, there's a noise in my room."*

After each call, Mom and I talked at length. "Don't you know that's the phone ringing? *"I never heard that before."* How come you're afraid of the phone? It wasn't the ring that startled her, although, on occasion, it did.

On my previous visits to her home, I spent several minutes clearing the answering machine, flooded with messages from telemarketers and those irritating robo calls. The ring was a nuisance she no longer tolerated; embarrassed she couldn't understand what was being asked of her. Mom always screened her calls, so the idea that thirty messages remained on her phone in a week didn't come as a surprise until now. On those occasions she did answer, she'd slam the phone in its cradle with enough force to crack the hard plastic covering.

Another source of Mom's angst with the phone was her inability to recognize the voices of those closes to her. For those people she could distinguish, Mom feared getting involved in conversation where someone might ask about a topic from the past.

Mom told no one she suffered from memory loss leaving that unenviable task to me. She didn't realize they already knew. Admitting any deficiency, in Mom's eyes is a monumental sign of weakness and embarrassment, neither tolerable. Even if she wanted to explain, she couldn't, Alzheimer's rendered her communications skills rudimentary at best when it came to complicated matters requiring more than superficial thought. A year latter, that phone is no longer in her room.

CHAPTER EIGHT

Discovery

Week 3 --- Mother's Day arrived long before its annual swing through the May calendar, but then again, everyday is now Mother's Day for us, she requires so much special attention.

Despite the fact we simplified Mom's wardrobe, she removes every stitch of clothing from her closet and lays them on the bed. She's done that each and every morning the previous two weeks.

"What should I wear pumpkin?" Wardrobe selection is serious business for Mom. *"Those don't match do they pumpkin?"* *"What color is this pumpkin,"* allowing Rusty to exam the fabric of her blouse with his damp nose.

Back and forth she goes, matching several blouses to a single pair of blue jeans. After twenty minutes, she closes the bedroom door and dresses.

When the door reopened, she got busy hanging or folding and refolding. My mind drifted back to my grandmother five years earlier, and her late night folding exercise. Not satisfied, she restarted the process several times before we intervened. I was so enmeshed in the battle of the outfits I'd forgotten I told Mom to take a shower.

Recognizing the next part would be equally as arduous, I turned on her shower and tested the temperature, splashed liquid soap on her washcloth, and reviewed with Mom where everything was located. She stood peering through the bathroom door at a safe distance. Something frightened her. Mom asked multiple redundant questions before she deemed it safe to enter.

She cautiously pulled back the shower curtain to make certain water indeed flowed from the faucet. Then she looked behind the bathroom door satisfying her curiosity that nothing lurked out of view that could possibly cause harm. Mom's confusion and apprehension lasted so long, like the previous shower steam obscured the bathroom mirror, mist drifting through the adjoining rooms.

Next came the battle of the soap. She couldn't reconcile the liquid body soap I put on her washcloth with the bar soap she used throughout her life. To my knowledge, she'd never used liquid bath soap, something so simple, yet so foreign to Mom. *"Is that really soap?"* I turned the plastic bottle upside down and squeezed a couple of drops into her hand. *"That smells good."*

Later that same afternoon came Mom's monthly hair appointment; only she hadn't set foot in the salon for at least three months. Her gray hair, caked with toothpaste she'd mistakenly applied as gel, made her mane stand up like a troll doll, akin to that of former boxing promoter Don King.

Mom used the same hairdresser for nearly ten years. Like most good stylists, they develop a bond with their clients, the customer often sharing intimate details of their lives as if sitting in a confessional. This relationship was no exception. I mentioned the name of her beautician several times before our arrival. *"Who?"* Names were now added to the list of things Mom no longer recognized. She needs a face to attach to a name, or the name itself is meaningless.

The sight of her stylist brought a surplus of tears and happiness. The two embraced, Mom holding on for dear life, forcing the hairdresser to gently release Mom's grip. The beautician knew of her condition and proved herself a good steward of Mom's emotions and feelings.

When I returned, they were listening to some old school R & B, sounding like two high school girls. Mom enjoyed the magic carpet ride back in time to the only part of her memory still partially intact, childhood in Atlantic City.

My grandmother owned a hair salon business in Atlantic City during Mom's youth. Maybe it was the smell of hot curling irons, shampoo, hair dyes, and hot dryers that stimulated a memory. Whatever took Mom back to 1957, the music or the smells, I'm uncertain, but it felt so familiar, I swear she'd gone back to high school, bobby socks and all.

Every time Mom visited her hairdresser, the reaction was equally heartfelt and memorable; the tight embrace of an old friend she hadn't seen in years, not realizing it had only been three weeks. A visit to the salon was worth the trouble, even if her stylist never touched a hair on her head.

* * *

Preparing Mom for bed typically took at least an hour. It usually started with taking Rusty for his nightly constitution. The little guy had the routine down cold. After returning with Rusty, I would fill up Mom's special water bottle, with the words WATER printed with a black sharpie on the side. I placed the bottle on her nightstand. Mom refused to consider sleep without the security of a water bottle nearby. Knowing she wouldn't find the bottle in the middle of the night, I placed it on her nightstand and made a spectacle of its position.

She examined the bottle carefully before acceptance. *"Are you sure that's water?"* she'd often ask. She would repeat the water bottle exam, spying it closely in the see-through pink container. "Mom that's water." *"Oh, I didn't know that was water."* Then she'd place the bottle in a precise location on her nightstand, like it had a pre-designated spot. She'd fidget with the location until satisfied it looked just right---another epic ritual that could easily last ten minutes.

Then came the constant reminder for her to change into nightclothes. She got in the habit of putting her pajamas on the shelf in the bedroom closet one day, the next, folded neatly in a drawer---a different drawer each time. She never remembered, so we searched for the buried treasure that was her pajamas. After weeks of pajama roulette, I would find them on my own without asking for her participation.

My approach to Mom was different than my girlfriend's. She demanded action, leaving no room for ambiguity or discussion. "Anita time to put your pajamas on," in a tone of voice I couldn't imagine being effective for me. Mom reacted like an elementary school student in the principal's office, about to receive punishment under the threat of calling your parents. Those pajamas were on in thirty seconds.

It would be some time before Mom reacted to my more soothing approach to this, and many other tasks. Mom hated being scolded like a little child, and at times would react in anger to my fiancé's commands, but even I had to admit, the drill sergeant approach could be effective, even for me, if used sparingly.

Mom had a habit of reading books in bed, falling asleep to the sound of a television before the onset of Alzheimer's. It's a part of her that survived post diagnosis. Tonight, Mom had her bible open on the nightstand, a book of affirmations resting open on the pillow next to her, and one of those trashy romance novels she'd read several years earlier in her hand.

Despite my exhaustion, having not slept for the better part of three days, I decided to leave Mom for a few minutes to enjoy her books. I watched quietly as she went back and forth between each book, once again mouthing the words. She paused after each sentence, reflecting, before reading the next. Mom caught me looking, smiled, and went back to digesting the contents of her books. The look she gave me reminded me of my own youth when I sought parental approval and con-firmation.

Once she tired of the books, Mom asked me, repeatedly, where the bathroom was located, fearful she couldn't find it once we went to bed. *"Maybe I'd better go now, just in case."* Since her gallbladder removal, Mom developed an obsession with using the restroom. It's an infatuation that borders on paranoia, with, or without Alzheimer's as the catalyst.

Then she'd turn to Rusty, *"You have to go to the bathroom pumpkin?"* Rusty would give that quizzical turn of the head like he didn't want to be bothered. He wouldn't budge, frustrating Mom. I finally stepped in; "Mom I just took Rusty out he's fine for the evening.*"* *"I didn't see him go, I'm the mommy, I have to see my DOOGIE go."* (Yes she pronounced it that way, always had) "It's okay mom, he's good for the night." *"But I need to see my dog go to make sure."* "Mom," in my slightly agitated voice, "he's not going anymore tonight, lets go to bed."

I set the television for automatic shutoff after three hours, turned on the Game Show Network, to *Family*

Feud, and started to leave the room when she stopped and asked what I'd done to her television. She wanted to know about the auto shutoff function. I explained it to her in language better suited for a two-year-old. *"I didn't know you could do that,"* came the satisfied reply of the mom child, *"that's cool."* I closed the door and collapsed on the living room sofa.

* * *

On advice from my aunt, we started giving Mom simple tasks, hoping to provide a distraction and build a little self-confidence. Today, it would be folding clean clothes.

When she completed that task, Mom emptied an entire box of tissues on her bed. She tore each tissue in half and proceeded to fold them into nice neat squares. She stacked the folded tissues in the top drawer of her nightstand, fussing over the precise location inside.

The following day, she repeated the tissue fold, emptying her drawer, and refolding those she'd so meticulously arranged the day before. If her supply ran low, Mom made sure I brought her a new box. It's a routine she performed with the utmost care making certain the stack wouldn't fall over.

* * *

We ate a huge dinner of chicken, rice, potatoes, and vegetables around 5:30 p.m., followed by ice cream.

Mom was fully engaged in conversation while we ate, laughing and joking. She looked really happy. Satisfied, she went to her room for more mindless television.

The quiet lasted just a few minutes when she burst into the kitchen complaining of hunger, clutching her stomach as if she were protecting a fetus from harm. When we informed her of the recently completed meal, she accused both of us of lying in a violent outburst of indignation. She became increasingly agitated. *"No, I didn't eat all of that,"* slamming her fist on the kitchen counter---her favorite act of defiance. *"That was hours ago."* We produced the meal calendar showing Mom what she consumed and then pointed at the clock. *"Why don't I remember?"*

I decided to step in and take advantage of the opportunity to explain her condition in the simplest terms possible. She sought answers. Ignoring her at this critical juncture didn't seem like the right thing to do, although a voice inside me said tread cautiously.

I went over Alzheimer's without using medical terms or large vocabulary. Mom concentrated on each word as it left my mouth. It appeared she was lip reading. She didn't want to miss a single detail. I went through a list of famous people who suffered from dementia.

I asked if she'd heard of President Reagan, whose beloved wife Nancy had just passed days earlier. There seemed to be a hint of recognition. I mentioned the former president for two reasons. It was far enough in the past that I thought it would trigger a memory.

Second, during her days of work at the Air Force Academy, President Reagan's picture was everywhere. Like most military installations, the current commander-in-chief's photo is prominently displayed next to, maybe the secretary of defense, the secretary of the Air Force and the current commander at the military installation assigned. I explained to Mom, how President Reagan had suffered like she suffered now.

"Is there a cure, I don't want to be like this?" Mom interrogated me better than a good lawyer. The foggy memory for the moment had disappeared. The questions were well thought out exactly as one would expect from someone in control of their mind. It appeared we were experiencing one of those great flashes of lucidity. I seized the opportunity knowing it could disappear any minute.

While I'd read numerous studies the past few weeks, none offered a cure in time for her, but that would be my secret. "Mom, they are rushing to find a cure." *"I hope so, I don't want to be like this,"* she repeated a few more times.

I decided to tread into deeper waters going over all her previous quarterly visits to the Cleveland Clinic. She had no recollection of those visits, a symptom of the short-term memory loss associated with Alzheimer's.

I decided to conduct my own informal memory exam because she was so alert and responsive. I started in reverse chronological order with her last job before retirement, approximately ten years earlier. I already knew she didn't remember anything about Las Vegas.

"Mom, do you remember Ft. Huachuca in Arizona?" My inquiry was greeted with the Alzheimer's Process Look, the question falling on a blank spot in her memory. "How about Sierra Vista, Arizona, do you remember that?" Sierra Vista is the home of Ft. Huachuca. *"It sounds vaguely familiar."*

Mom worked at Ft. Huachuca for over a decade as a computer technician, a job she was forced into for career advancement. Despite her schooling and other training, she'd often call me at home to explain when she had a problem, knowing my Air Force job involved computers. I repeated her home street address in Sierra Vista. She remembered the sequence of numbers, but not the street.

I went back to the Air Force Academy, and the Colorado Springs area where she lived for twenty years. We arrived as a nuclear family in 1974. A lot happened to our family at the Academy. All three of Mom's children graduated from high school. My parents' divorced. She bought two homes. Her career blossomed, taking on the first of many supervisory roles. One of her best friends from those Academy years' lives just two miles from her current house in Las Vegas. The wormhole had opened wide sucking forty years of memories into a dimension of the brain she couldn't access, or those cells were simply dead.

Then she blurted out, *"I worked for the military my entire life."* I confirmed her recollection, "yes Mom, that's right, you did," in a voice that might have sounded condescending to an adult in full control of their faculties.

I decided to go back four more years, to our arrival at Tyndall Air Force Base, in Panama City, Florida, in 1970. We lived at Tyndall for four years. I mentioned the Gulf of Mexico and her work at the Base Exchange shoe store. She always asked vendors to deliver size 13 shoes for her tall lanky son. If anything would trigger a memory at Tyndall, it would be my shoe size. My feet were the butt of so many jokes in our community, not a week went by where someone didn't make fun of Daffy Duck feet in her presence. Mom often led the charge. My retelling the story never found a receptacle.

"Mom, do you remember Loring Air Force Base, in northern Maine? Remember how much it snowed there and how cold it was? Remember that's where Dad taught you how to drive a car? Remember your youngest daughter was born there?" *"Whose my daughter?"* I'd now gone back fifty years, nothing.

Ok, I tried one more test. "Mom do you remember living in Madrid, Spain?" *"Is that across the ocean?"* "Yes, yes," I shouted. Details of our three years in Madrid were fleeting, but at least she remembered something. I reminded her of our maid Consuelo, who taught me Spanish, and my elementary school years. She knew the maid's name and had a vague recollection of walking me to the school bus.

I should have stopped here, but curiosity got the better of me. I pried even deeper and mentioned Atlantic

City, New Jersey. *"When can we go home,"* she asked, thinking she was that little girl of the 1940s and 50s.

She morphed into a trip down memory lane all on her own. She talked about the house on the corner. It was Mom's home prior to the one she lived in at my birth. She described the neighborhood in fine detail. It was a home I knew nothing about. I asked my aunt a few weeks later about that house and discovered Mom's recollection to be true down to the finest detail.

She talked about the Boardwalk, her mother being a former hairdresser, and St. James AME Church.

The memories of Atlantic City were so vivid---her eyes, body language, voice, every element of her being came alive in a heightened state of awareness. I was shocked at the detailed recollection.

In fifteen minutes, we'd observed multiple versions of the same person, easily slipping from moments of great confusion, to clarity, and back to confusion.

"Do you remember meeting Dad in Atlantic City?" *"Who?"* "Dad, Richard Bennett. How did you get your last name?" *"I don't remember him."*

My parent's married shortly after high school and remained husband and wife for over twenty years. It was his career that led her to travel the country and carried us to Spain.

This nightmarish horror script of lost memories is something I couldn't write just a few short years ago, and now this movie played out before my eyes in unending agony. It's a script that unfortunately could not be rewritten with a happier ending. I desperately wanted to reach her so I tried one more test. "Do you remember attending Church of God in Christ here in Las Vegas? You went every Sunday with your best friend."

"My mother sang in the choir and played the piano. I don't know why she (her mother) made me sing in that choir, I had no business in anybody's choir, not with my voice," as a sheepish grin of a well-delivered punch line to a joke crossed her face. I smiled, all while realizing Mom was back in Atlantic City. By now, I'm certain I'd thoroughly confused her with my fifty questions.

Just a split second after her self-deprecating humor, Mom became serious, frustrated by her inability to remember the past, except Atlantic City. Her brow furrowed trying really hard to remember something. Her eyes darted back and forth, staring at the kitchen table, then up at me, then down at the table again. I told her some day she would forget me too. Her eyes saddened at the thought, denying she would ever forget. It was a nice sentiment for sure, but one I knew not to be true, and deep down she believed I was correct in my assessment.

"Mom do you know how many children you have?" It was the fourth consecutive day I'd asked that question. This was the first day she gave me the correct answer, but the way she answered told me it was more a guess than a definitive statement.

I probably should've avoided so many attempts to trigger past memories, but I knew Mom would do almost anything to please me. Looking back, I now believe I was attempting to satisfy myself more than help her remember, I so desperately wanted my mother back.

I asked Mom to name her children. The only name she remembered was mine. Mom reached up and grabbed my hand in celebration like she just won the lottery.

In total, the conversation lasted more than an hour. I didn't want it to end, enjoying the repartee, but I knew I'd pushed further than prudence dictated. Taxing an Alzheimer's patient this much is dangerous territory.

Our evaluation of Mom's cognitive function continued at breakfast the following morning. She appeared fresh after a night of limited sleep, which meant the morning hours, presented an opportunity to have a relaxed discussion before the daily activity brought about confusion and hallucinations.

Mom typically didn't eat anything she couldn't recognize. We prepared a ham and egg omelet, added grapes, and an English muffin. Recognition of the grapes came easy. She identified the eggs as "first" boiled eggs and couldn't identify the ham, despite the fact, she'd eaten it her entire life.

We put strawberry jelly on the English muffin. Mom loved anything sweet, and remarked how much she enjoyed the muffin. "Mom, what's on your muffin? What is it that makes it sweet?" She thought hard for a minute, but couldn't identify the sweet sticky substance. For the next twenty minutes I told her about jelly and its many flavors. I had a knack for telling stories that she appreciated. She was salivating. Something about sweet and sticky hit a nerve. She talked about her favorite sweets---ice cream, lemon meringue pie and more.

I joked about my own insatiable appetite for peanut butter and jelly sandwiches during my youth. It wasn't uncommon for me to eat an entire loaf of bread at one sitting during my high school years. Mom scolded me often for my excessive eating habits. *"Next time you go and buy the bread,"* she'd yell, knowing full well that wouldn't happen. This was the true definition of gluttony. The next day my bread would be replaced with a new loaf.

At lunch we played "name the food." It took several minutes for Mom to identify rice. When she realized she'd given the correct answer, she applauded. Of course we played it up in our own celebratory way.

"Anita, what's that meat you're eating," my girlfriend asked? *"I don't know, but sure is good."* "Can you name some meats that you might have eaten in the past?" Is hamburger a meat?" *"I think so."*

"How about chicken, is that chicken you're eating a meat, Anita?" She looked at me to provide a clue. I remained motionless, trying to encourage her with my eyes; go ahead Mom, it's okay if you get the wrong answer. *"I think its meat."* We clapped and danced wildly around the room.

After lunch, we took Mom to see *Zootopia*. Yes, it was a children's movie, but I didn't want her first experience with us to be a dark movie, a mystery, or a thriller. Following complex or highly emotional storylines caused Mom a great deal of distress. Our choice of entertainment turned into a blessing. The characters were cute and some of the jokes were easy to understand. Sitting in that darkened theater made me appreciate the therapeutic affects of music on dementia sufferers. She bounced around in her seat like a kid on a sugar high.

Once home, having observed such a powerfully positive change in demeanor, we placed our spare radio in her room. Mom is a music genre agnostic---she'd listen to everything from R & B to country, as long as it had a beat, or easy to follow lyrics with a nice melody.

The radio was a Bose that turned on with a single swipe of the hand across the top---no buttons to push. I thought this would be an easy lesson. I opened the palm of my hand and slid it across the top in one smooth motion. I repeated the motion to turn the radio off. "You try it," I said. She punched at the top of the radio with her fist, growing increasingly frustrated at the silence.

I gently grabbed her arm by the wrist and had her open her hand, palm down. Together we swiped her hand across the top. She fell in lockstep with an old Diana Ross and the Supremes song she recognized. When the song finished, Mom started punching at the radio once again, this time palm open. The radio just played on.

Once again, I demonstrated with my own hand, then held hers to try again. After thirty minutes, I gave up. "I will turn the radio on and off for you." *"Good, I don't want to break anything,"* satisfied I'd solved some major crisis.

* * *

What is it about music and lyrics the allows Mom to remember songs fifty and sixty years old, but she can't recall what occurred in her life yesterday?

Countless studies suggest music, when used appropriately can, "shift mood, manage stress-induced agitation, stimulate positive interactions, facilitate cognitive function, and coordinate motor skills." The above quote came from a story I found on the Alzheimer's Foundation website.

My mother, and many other Alzheimer's patients I've observed respond so positively to music, we've made it a major part of Mom's life. When we're in the car, I make sure the radio is on and keep conversation to a minimum. Her mind is gone to another dimension, where I have no clue, but it's vastness is one filled with warmth and excitement with music as the backdrop.

Even in the quiet of the car, Mom sings loudly, reciting the lyrics as if she wrote them herself. I've never witnessed such an immediate and complete transformation in mood and attitude. At home, she sits in a music-induced coma for hours while folding her tissues.

My first clue to the power of music was the Christmas party at the assisted living center a few months earlier. The gentleman who performed that evening invited Mom to the stage where she remained singing and dancing for an hour, never once compelled to rest.

Music is magic. "It can spark compelling outcomes even in very late stages of Alzheimer's and related dementias." Play a song my mother recognizes, at times she'll be motivated to dance ignoring the pain in her joints. Mom often grabs Rusty by his front paws and moves him about mimicking some dance move she remembers.

"This happens because rhythmic and other well-rehearsed responses require little to no cognitive or mental processing. They are influenced by the motor center of the brain that responds directly to auditory rhythmic clues. A person's ability to engage in music, particularly rhythm playing and singing, remains intact late into the disease process because, again, these activities do not mandate cognitive functioning for success."

"Most people associate music with important events and a wide array of emotions. The connection can be so strong that hearing a tune long after the occurrence evokes a memory of it."

Stimulative music activates while sedative music quiets. Think about your own lives. When I'm at the gym, I'm usually listening to some music with increased tempo, especially when engaged in intense cardio. During my evening hours, or when I'm in the car alone, it's a nice ballad for relaxation. My mother has similar moments of expression.

The story on the Alzheimer's website suggests those in late stage Alzheimer's could suffer from auditory overload and become agitated if you choose the wrong music, one with heavy metal beats, or increased tempo.

For our mother, music puts her in a catatonic state oblivious to the outside world for hours after the music has vanished.

To read the complete story about music or other care related stories, go to the Alzheimer's Foundation website alzfdn.org and look under the link for Caregiving Resources.

* * *

We were now less than a month away from that scheduled business trip out of the country. To prepare for Amanda's arrival, I labeled all the family photos in Mom's room. The only photos she recognized without thought were her parents'. I tagged photos of my sister and her daughter, with their names and the caption, "your youngest daughter" and "your granddaughter."

I put Mom's best friend's photo above her phone, since it was she who called most often. I labeled my son's photo, Karen's photo, along with Mom's brother and both sisters'. Everyday, I quizzed her. Even with the labels, she got things mixed up in her head, but I often caught her staring at those pictures, reciting the names under her breath.

I decided to remove all the labels except Mandi's and my niece to make it easier, since they were the ones planning to watch her during our time away.

We increased the frequency of Skype calls to breed more familiarity. I'd told Mom a few days earlier that we'd be gone a week. The mention of our time away created an anxiety-inducing event that left her visibly shaken. *"What's going to happen to me? I don't want to be here alone."* I decided right then and there not to mention it again.

I remained concerned my sister still didn't know what she signed up for, and how far Mom's disease had progressed. She spoke to Mom like she retained most of her memory. Despite my previous request not to mention the trip, my sister brought the subject to Mom's attention, eliciting a frightful reaction that forced me to terminate the call.

I wanted to scream, but opted to explain how Alzheimer's worked. Mom's mind is her tomb. She's trapped in a reality that changes from minute to minute. I realized after numerous conversations, no amount of explanation from me could adequately convey Mom's reality. Alzheimer's care had to be experienced. I just needed to soften the blow.

During conversations with my sister, I found myself dictating terms of communications with her own mother. Do this, don't do that, watch out for this, keep Mom on a consistent schedule, give her medications at this time of day, record all of Mom's meals, don't leave toothpaste in the bathroom Mom thinks it's hair gel, put the child-locks on all kitchen cabinets and the refrigerator---my list of directions forced me to create a bible of care for Mom, one that Mandi could easily follow.

* * *

As the end of week three approached, we decided a trip to the park was in order. Walking is ingrained in Mom from her youth in Atlantic City. Her family never owned a car. Need to go to the grocery story, you walked and carried the heavy bags home. My grandmother used a two-wheeled steel-framed folding grocery basket for just such occasions. Time to go to church, you walked, school a combination of pounding the pavement and the bus. Trips to the Boardwalk, you walked---the Hicks car was your feet. Inclement weather mattered little. Mom didn't even learn how to drive a car until age twenty-six. My grandfather's open-road driving was limited to his experience during World War II as far as I know.

When we arrived at the park with Rusty, the outdoor air fostered an awakening in Mom of a dormant past. Rusty bolted at the thought of freedom, before his leash snapped him back a few paces. He eventually settled into a routine of running ahead of Mom, then waiting for her to catch up. He seldom got more than twenty paces in front of her. If Mom didn't arrive quickly enough at Rusty's rendezvous point, he backtracked to meet her.

Mom spoke nonstop of Atlantic City while we walked two laps around the dirt-laden track that formed the park's boundaries. The interior was a beautiful green, with rolling hills, three picnic tables, lots of trees, several tennis courts, and a playground for young kids. *"We walked every where. My parents' didn't own a car,"* she exclaimed, proud she'd gotten so far on her feet. She repeated herself no fewer than a half dozen times that first lap. She either forgot she'd mentioned it previously or was attempting to start a conversation after long moments of silence. We just listened, letting her revel in happy days gone by.

She noticed the birds chirping and the solitude of our surroundings. *"Those houses look just like ours in Atlantic City."* I don't know what symphony played inside Mom's head, but these large Las Vegas Mediterranean style stucco homes look nothing like the typical Atlantic City walkup. No need correcting her; just let the band play on. Our conversations seemed so adolescent at times, like that of a precocious child.

After the walk, we sat at picnic tables enjoying the other dogs at play. One gentleman played Frisbee with a small German Sheppard running freely through the park's rolling hills. Rusty went ballistic, barking nonstop. Mom tried to hush Rusty, but he was having none of it, until he wanted to quit. Rusty wasn't accustomed to outdoor spaces he had to share with other dogs. After a few minutes he quieted down and watched the German Sheppard catch the Frisbee and run back to its owner.

Mom gazed skyward at the contrails left by planes from several nearby airports. It reminded me of my youth, lying on the grass looking up at the clouds with my friends. "Hey that cloud looks like an camel." "That one has two eyes looking at us." Mom had no clouds on this day, but the planes captured her imagination with youthful exuberance. Despite her fear of flying, she'd always been fascinated by planes. I just assumed it was an extension of our lives growing up on Air Force bases. In Florida, fighter jets buzzed our house around 6 a.m., six days a week rousting my sisters' and me out of bed in time for school.

* * *

Once home, Mom ate lunch and started working her puzzle with renewed enthusiasm. She'd ignored the puzzle for the better part of a week. I guess the fresh air cleared her jumbled mind. An hour passed when she bolted from her room to ask, *"Can we put the puzzle in a picture frame and hang it on the wall when we're done?"* It was a beautiful memory from her past that pulled at my heartstrings. I was reminded of the days when our family had few material possessions, relying on the love of our mother to sustain us.

CHAPTER NINE

School In Session

eek 4 --- It started like any other since Mom's arrival, that is until I entered her room early one morning. The strong smell of urine interrupted the lilac room freshener from the adjoining room.

At first, I thought Rusty had an accident. I checked the carpet, the floor, the bedding, and found nothing. I looked for clues in Rusty's behavior, knowing he'd be embarrassed at the thought he messed up, there were none.

I was disgusted at myself for even thinking Mom might have wet herself, she'd never done that before. After exhausting the Rusty options I discreetly checked Mom's bedding and night clothing, she too was dry.

By now, Rusty is barking his intense displeasure at me for having made him wait so long before taking him outside. Okay little guy, "lets go," I said, still no closer to the source of the pungent odor.

Upon my return, I continued the search while Mom headed for the restroom. I checked the closet and bedding once again, before I spotted the source---the small wastebasket in the corner. How in the hell did she manage to relieve herself in the trashcan? I quietly emptied the contents before her return, knowing she would deny peeing in the can, or embarrassed at the thought she might have.

Still speechless at my discovery, I called Karen. "You wouldn't believe it, Mom pissed in the trashcan." *"What, she never did that here."* My sister's response got me to thinking. Did fear and paranoia at unfamiliar surroundings trap her inside the room?

Maybe I was culpable. Mom drank so little water over the years I'm surprised her veins hadn't collapsed. After our walk the previous day, I told her to drink a big bottle of water. She did exactly as I asked. The combination of too much water and new environment might have created a situation she couldn't reconcile. At least she used the trashcan, although, for the life of me, I physically don't know how.

I removed all liquid from her room after 7 p.m., allowing only a sip of water with medicine. I made her use the facilities before bed. I gave her the quiz, each and every night before lights out. "Mom show me where the bathroom is." "Can you find the bathroom"? The bathroom is right outside her bedroom door. Each time I quizzed her, she gave me that "do you think I'm stupid look."

Satisfied, I went to bed, waking the next morning to a urine free room. In the five months that followed, she's only missed the bathroom two other times, once about a week later.

* * *

No matter how late I went to bed, or how early I woke, Mom always appeared to be stirring. If I went to bed at 1 a.m., she was awake. If I rose before the crack of dawn, Mom was awake. At no time did it appear she ever slept for more than an hour at a time, nor would she take a nap during the day any longer.

We thought about putting a baby monitor in her room, to better understand her sleep habits. I wanted one with a camera, but thought it violated what little privacy and dignity she had remaining.

Rusty slept more than Mom and would announce his displeasure if roused too early. Mom's face provided a telltale sign of whether she had a fitful nights sleep. The bags under her eyes most mornings looked like she'd gone ten rounds with a heavy weight boxer. In our case the reigning champ was the undefeated Alzheimer's. Mom could be downright hostile without sleep, completely paradoxical to her normal behavior.

My girlfriend's mother mentioned reading about Alzheimer's patients receiving sleep medication from their doctors. I did my own little research and found websites touting the effectiveness of sleeping aids for Devil's Disease sufferers. Many of the prescribed medications seemed rather addictive, which raised a red flag. For me, any medication is a last resort.

Other sites suggested less habit-forming measures such as melatonin or moderate exercise to tire out the Alzheimer's patient. We'd already started the exercise and that did nothing to induce sleep.

* * *

This from Neurology Now magazine April/May 2016. *Sleep Smarter* by Marisa Cohen.

"Deep, uninterrupted slumber is important for everyone, but it's especially critical for people with neurologic disorders. Sleep deprivation can make symptoms such as pain, stiffness, memory loss, fatigue, and confusion worse and can provoke seizures and headaches. Here's the rub, though: the very disorder that make sleep such a valued commodity are responsible for robbing you of the rest you need...The 'body clock' that controls wake-sleep cycles is located in the hypothalamus" portion of the brain." "...for people with neurologic conditions such as Alzheimer's disease, the internal clock can become completely unplugged."

According to Dr. Jennifer Molano, MD FAAN, associate professor of neurology at the University of Cincinnati,

"In studies of people with Alzheimer's disease, we can see disease-related changes in that part of the brain (hypothalamus), which can be associated with an irregular sleep-wake cycle. In fact, there is evidence that sleep disturbances goes both ways: amyloid plaques, hallmarks of Alzheimer's disease, affect the brain, altering sleep cycles; and lack of sleep promotes the creation and spread of the plaques."

So what does all this mean? In a nutshell, those amyloid plaques, one of the main causes of Alzheimer's are made worse by lack of sleep, yet it's the very lack of sleep that creates and spreads the plaques, destroying the brain and its sleep centers.

No one epitomizes this phenomenon better than our mother. We've tried several treatments to induce sleep, some you'll read about later. None of them have been effective. I honestly don't know how she functions, and remain amazed she hasn't hurt herself or attempted to wander off. We've given up pushing hardcore sleep, willing to settle for just resting on a schedule of our choosing. To date, its worked allowing us to sleep with one eye open.

* * *

I spent most of my free moments contemplating relocation back to Southern California where most of my business interests remain. I want Mom near me, whether in a memory care facility or in-home care with a twenty-four-hour nurse had yet to be determined.

I called a memory care facility in one of the beach communities near my old house. I spoke to a pleasant woman for nearly an hour going over Mom's state of mind and determining the level of care required. I explained the pee in the trash incident and was told to expect more of the same.

Now for the numbers: "We charge $225 a day, or $7,650 a month," she said. That is $4,000 more than Mom's pension and social security combined. The air rushed from my lungs as I ran those figures through my head. I recovered quickly to ask what the costs covered. I already knew the answer; I just needed a moment to process the jolt to my system.

I must not have feigned shock well enough. The memory care representative told me she had another option I should consider. "I don't know what your living situation will be at home, but your mom can come here from 6 a.m. to 6 p.m. daily. We charge $125 a day for memory care, but you'd still need a nighttime nurse if you don't want to take care of your Mom when she becomes incontinent." Well thanks for nothing I thought to myself. Mom's income covered Monday through Friday daycare only. Weeknights and weekends were another matter entirely, and one I knew she couldn't afford.

Defeated, for the moment, I graciously accepted her offer to send me additional information with the promise to stay in touch and hung up. I sat motionless. Nothing prepared me for that collision---the prohibitive cost versus my expectations. I shouldn't have been surprised by now, but I just couldn't reconcile the expense. Why so costly, and why weren't there adequate financial resources to mitigate this expense?

* * *

I looked down at Rusty. He seemed lethargic. He barked at me, signaling time for a potty break. We made it outside just in time as he defecated everywhere. Great, now he was sick. My first thoughts went to what had Mom fed him out of sight of our watchful eyes.

We later discovered Mom snuck food into a napkin, slid the contents into her nightstand drawer, and either closed the door, or waited until we went to sleep. Then Rusty feasted on whatever non-dog delicacy she provided.

Rusty continued emptying his little system after we returned. Mom screamed, *"What's happening to my dog?"* Once Rusty finished, he hid in fear behind Mom's leg under the table. Rusty knew not to use the bathroom indoors, and thought he'd committed a mortal sin. It took awhile before I coaxed him from under the table and reassured my little buddy we weren't upset.

In fact, we were upset, and maybe he sensed it, but not at him. We discovered Mom's food stash and decided right then and there to use it as a teachable moment, hoping beyond hope that part of it would stick. Of one thing we were certain, Mom would never intentionally hurt Rusty, he was her rock. We hammered home the theme of not feeding Rusty, other than his own food.

"You see what just happened to him?" We were scolding her like a child. She felt awful; I could see it in her eyes. We made her read the sign on the table "DON'T FEED RUSTY!" Five months later that sign remains, but Rusty has not had another bite of Mom's food.

* * *

We began to notice a very distinct behavioral pattern, occurring daily between 3 p.m. and 5 p.m. The cumulative effects of the day's events seem to wear Mom down creating a heightened state of confusion. While she paces often throughout the day, this time slot brings with it a more deliberative walk, a frenetic like pace between her bedroom and the balcony.

The Alzheimer's Stare, the vacant eyes, and a face that shows lack of sleep, leads to behavior that often manifests itself through constantly challenging authority, primarily mine. At first, I ignored the behavior, until it reached a point where I feared she might injure herself. And honestly, it annoyed the hell out of me.

Screaming she hadn't eaten all day, Mom chose this time to attempt to prepare a meal, despite having just eaten within the past hour. Knowing the severity of her gastrointestinal problems, I couldn't allow her to eat so soon, or she'd be writhing in pain.

We quickly intervened, but Mom's inability to accept reason and compromise rendered any attempts to calm her down useless. Mom slammed her fist on the counter, then turned and pounded the side of the refrigerator hard enough to leave a small indentation. The moment had the potential of turning violent, requiring me to get a little more heavy-handed than I would have preferred.

At my size, any deliberate move on my part could be quite intimidating to a woman so small in stature. I grabbed Mom, rather forcefully by both her wrist. *"Get your hands off of me,"* she screamed in a demonic voice that would have made Linda Blair from *The Exorcist* movie fame proud.

Knowing, she'd attack if I let go, I held tight. "Mom lets go to your room for a moment." *"Make me, make me, I dare you, I dare you, you guys are liars,"* the beast had arisen now at full fury. Had the neighbors been home, one of them, I'm certain would have called the police. She had daggers in her eyes, every sharp-edged sword piercing my body a thousand times over. She'd gone berserk.

I released a little pressure on her wrist, thinking she'd meet me halfway, and refrain from striking back. She had other ideas and tried valiantly to pull away, fist wrapped tight ready to strike. When I reapplied the pressure she quickly realized I meant business. To satisfy her urge to lash out, she resorted to taunts and kicks, one landing on poor Rusty's rear-end, the other, a glancing blow to my shin.

I pulled Mom across the kitchen floor to her bedroom. Resistance for her would have been futile at that point. I sat her on the bed. She continued the taunts and threats upon my body before I decided to use my booming drill sergeant voice. "MOM, KNOCK IT OFF." The room went quiet. She crossed a line. This dangerous behavior needed to stop. My voice was all I had left in my arsenal. I slowly released the pressure on her wrist.

Thirty minutes from start to finish, it was all over. She had returned to normal, in a true Dr. Jekyll and Mr. Hyde moment. Unfortunately, this incident would be one of many in the weeks and months ahead. Fortunately, none rose to the level of violence of this first episode. I've since adjusted my approach to her moving target of emotions and behaviors, trying my best to stay in front of any potential conflict.

The following morning I bounced into Mom's room like every morning to give her medicine before breakfast. The fear in her eyes told me she retained a piece of the ugliness from the day before. She acted as if I were about to spank her. In her mind the incident happened moments ago, when in reality it had been a good eighteen hours. I sat with her knowing she needed the loving son's reassurance. I told her I loved her, kissed her forehead, and took Rusty out for a walk.

* * *

I saw the phrase "Sundowning" during one of the many applications I filled out for assistance. I actually left that block on the form blank the first time, waiting to ask an intake coordinator at a memory care facility the meaning. "It's late day disorientation and confusion," she said, "that could cause severe behavioral changes."

The universe could indeed be a strange place, how else to explain Mom's bizarre behavior the day before. So I asked more questions. "What does it do?" "How is it treated?" "Is it the same time everyday?" "Does it have to do with the sun setting?" She answered with as much specificity as she could, but the counselor wasn't a doctor. She dealt with the abhorrent behavior after the fact.

Mom's late afternoon, child like tirades usually occur between 3 p.m. and 5 p.m. Not exactly sunset, but definitely an accumulation of a days worth of activities with little to no sleep. The rants typically last approximately thirty minutes. When she exhibited her first tantrum, I was uncertain it fit the classic definition of sundowners, but the consistency, along with the counselor's comments, sure made it seem like it fit the pattern.

One of the triggers was our refusal to continually provide food. Mom would fall on the floor, pound her fists on the nearest piece of furniture and scream uncontrollably. The screams were typically incoherent rants of a child, aimed once again at me. She would look at Rusty and say, *"come on, we're getting out of here, these people don't care about us."* I fell for the act the first few times, before I determined it to be a ruse for attention. Minutes later, like before, she had no recollection of the tantrum.

The other, more serious trigger had a time element to it that coincided with her gastrointestinal attacks, real and perceived, regardless of time of day. Mom had become so conditioned to stomach problems over the years she often acted out of anticipation, rather than the real event.

Unlike the gastrointestinal attacks earlier in the day, where she would managed the pain until it passed, these late afternoon outbursts were ugly and violent. Mom would throw her body on the floor, landing with a loud thud, arms flailing about. I tried to pick her up once. She screamed, *"You're hurting me,"* as I lightly place my hands under her elbows to provide leverage. These eruptions were alarming and only occurred at home.

I'm convinced, even without scientific evidence to the contrary; her gastrointestinal attacks are a side effect of Alzheimer's. Nothing in her history suggests these attacks are associated with normal digestion, the types of food she eats, or the time of her last meal.

* * *

I felt myself getting enraged by the day. My emotions were under assault. My career goals and objectives were losing to providing for my mother, yet, I needed a serious increase in income to support what could be a lengthy illness, if DNA can be used as a guide. I read tons of literature and research suggesting most Alzheimer's patients were dead within eight years of diagnosis. It seems obvious to me that Mom will make the eight-year threshold with room to spare.

It was during this research I saw Alzheimer's referred to as the "Devil's Disease" for the first time. Satan already had a firm unrelenting grasp on Mom's mind. No amount of prayer could reverse the damage already done, yet, I held out hope, knowing the odds were against us; that's me, ever the eternal optimist.

People died from complications of Alzheimer's. Still naïve about the power of this disease, I couldn't comprehend what "death from complications of Alzheimer's" truly meant. Mom hadn't come close to exhibiting the more serious signs of death by Alzheimer's---the refusal to eat, aspiration pneumonia, failure of body systems, falls and broken bones.

But she had already shown her inability too basic problem solve and reason. The simplest of tasks now take twice as long to perform. Problems expressing thoughts, potentially violent behavior, the inability to sleep, fear, paranoia, limited hallucinations, and not recognizing family members are all indications of moderate stage sufferers; not death.

* * *

On the Sunday of our fourth week together, we were back to my fiancé's parents' home for our weekly

Sunday brunch. It would be the first time our parents' met. My girlfriend's family knew about Mom's illness, but like Mandi, they were about to discover, that no amount of intelligent conversation prepares you for Alzheimer's in real life. I never discussed how nervous I was about that dinner. Would Mom have a "sundowning" moment, or, be on her best behavior?

Brunch went better than expected, the devil allowing my real mother to shine through---always on her best behavior in public. It was a legacy left over from the teachings of her parents' who would never tolerate acting a fool in public, no matter the circumstances.

The only person more nervous than me that day was our cook, my future mother-in-law. She told me about those nerves before I used my warped sense of humor to diffuse the tension.

When we arrived, after the introductions, I took Mom to the patio while the food was being prepared. Our hosts' couldn't have been more gracious, clearing off the patio furniture so Mom could sit, offering her snacks and a bottle of water.

Mom was mesmerized, marveling at the peace and solitude of the tree-lined backyard on an eighty-five degree day. She commented about the quiet as her eyes settled on the beautiful landscaping silhouetted against the bright blue sky---the benefit of living in a senior citizens neighborhood far from the hustle and bustle of city life.

In her mind, she'd been whisked away to Atlantic City. The time travel machine dropped her off in high school sixty years earlier. She talked about the beach and the Boardwalk, describing certain landmarks and hotels that hadn't been around in decades. We sat quietly and listened, I only interjected to explain parts of Atlantic City to our hosts.

The call to eat woke Mom from her Atlantic City coma. At the table, she spoke when spoken to, but remained quiet throughout, her only complaint; *"I can't chew that,"* she whispered, referring to the brisket on her plate, which I'd already cut to the size of breadcrumbs. On a whim, I gave her a piece of my halibut, which she thoroughly enjoyed. Three pieces later, Mom was satisfied.

Showcasing her sweet tooth, Mom ate four mini pies and two bowls of ice cream before returning to the patio. No one witnessing that day would ever believe she had a debilitating neurologic disorder.

I took Mom home leaving my bride-to-be to enjoy quality time with her family. No sooner had we arrived, Mom started complaining she hadn't eaten. I quickly changed the subject and she never mentioned food again. I'd learned the fine art of beguiling and other forms of trickery to deflect most of her abhorrent behaviors.

Since we had such a good time with my girlfriend's family, I decided to reopen the laboratory to investigate Mom's mind. "Do you remember where we ate brunch?" *"No"* "Do you remember meeting the people who owned the house where we ate?" *"No"* "How about the four pies you ate, do you remember that?" A smile pursed her lips at the thought of the sweet stuff. That memory resonated when nothing else did. With that, I closed the lab allowing her to settle in and watch television.

* * *

Three thoughts occupied my mind as the first month drew to a close. First, we survived. I was no closer to long-term care solutions than the day Mom arrived, but we lived to fight another day.

My next thought, morbid as it is, had become an absolute necessity---what to do when Mom left us for heaven. I wanted this conversation years ago, before I got a front row seat to her declining health, but it wasn't in the cards. It's easier to confront these issues at a time when you think your loved one will live for all eternity.

Mom made no plans for funeral services, burial sites, and the financial burdens that come with such matters. It seemed most appropriate her remains should be in Atlantic City. Mom's love affair with this beach resort is indisputable.

Then I started thinking about cremation, a request my father made when he passed away. Would that appropriately honor my mother? I wallowed in self-pity thinking about the uncomfortable task at hand.

Then a more gruesome thought entered my subconscious, gruesome only to me, I guess, because I thought more about cutting Mom into tiny pieces if I donated her brain to science. I shuttered at the thought, sending my heart rate skyward for a few brief moments.

Then an equally devastating thought pushed cremation aside. What would happen if Rusty left us before Mom? It felt like a million volts of electricity coursed through my body. I felt the hair rise on the back of my hand and beads of sweat cascade down my forehead towards my brow.

Rusty already lived half his life expectancy of fourteen to sixteen years. I could only hope that if he left us before Mom, her memory would be so far gone she wouldn't notice, a prospect I thought unlikely. If the reverse were true, I'm not sure Rusty would survive. What a gloomy, morose few minutes of reflection.

Ironic how Alzheimer's now means Mom will never deal with what she'd avoided so long, those pesky details of late life decisions. It took every once of my being to refrain from blaming Mom for her selfishness. Her plan to fight off old age was never succumbing to the inevitable.

Her best friend mentioned to me, just days after Mom moved in, that Mom believed I would always take care of her. I felt so alone, not for dealing with Alzheimer's, my support system had started to take shape alleviating some emotional distress. Rather, it was the unwanted tough choices foisted upon me by the woman I loved more than any other, that created the chaos in my mind. It just didn't feel right making these decisions without her input. I vowed never to dump that burden on my son.

ACT 3

"Mem'ries,
Like the corners of my mind
Misty water-colored memories
Of the way we were"

The Way We Were
Sung by Barbra Streisand
Lyrics by Alan Bergman and Marilyn Bergman

CHAPTER TEN

What Now?

Next Six Months --- A monotonous routine took shape over the next few months, one I did not control---in fact, I hated what we'd become; caregivers. Virtually every waking juncture of my existence now swallowed whole by mommy obligations.

I learned several valuable lessons during my early teen years, to combat mounting frustration and confusion on life's labyrinth of twists and turns. I chastised myself more times than I could count for losing perspective over, what, in hindsight were trivial matters, allowing others to see my youthful explosive temper.

As I matured, I gained control of my emotions regardless of the serious nature of what lay before me. I prided myself on always being measured in my response to any crisis, preferring to retreat to the recesses of deep thought before responding. Like top professional athletes, I could channel the pressure of the moment into positive action. That wasn't happening this time. I fought to reject the bitterness and cynicism that now crept into my thoughts---my own battle of the mind.

The relationship with my girlfriend remained under constant assault. I kept a watchful eye, studying her facial expressions, and body language, listening carefully for the slightest tonal inflection that would provide evidence of her thoughts at any given moment. The tiniest sigh, roll of the eyes, or shake of the head would not go unnoticed. Then I would catch myself, thinking I might be too sensitive.

This beautiful creature is a proud, intelligent woman, as tough as they come. She wore her emotions for all to see, a byproduct of her Spanish and Puerto Rican heritage. Because she loved me, she tried valiantly to hide her angst, but I wasn't fooled.

Mom, on the other hand was blind to the turmoil her illness caused. After a month, she completely forgot her home of ten years; save for the moments she thought Rusty needed a bathroom break on our balcony.

The wild pendulum of Mom's memory was simply too inconsistent to predict. It typically swung hardest towards memory loss and stuck there for days, before making a rapid swing towards lucidity, then quickly returning to her detachment from reality. Each swing towards forgetfulness stuck and lasted longer than the previous journey.

We had numerous discussions with Mom over the next few weeks, usually precipitated by one of her temporary remembrances, or some flash of an idea that fixated itself in her conscious. Mom seemed to recognize that if she didn't speak her mind right then, she'd forget.

"Don't I have any family?" or *"Where is my family?"* were the two most difficult conversations to entertain. I never dodged those questions. I let her ask all the family questions she wanted, as often as she wanted. I didn't want Mom thinking she'd been abandoned, even if the worry were only temporary.

Each and every time she asked me about family, I would start with the numerous photo albums stored away in her bedroom. I'd bring them to the kitchen table and methodically go through each and every one. "Mom these are your two daughters." *"Where are they now?"* "California and Las Vegas." *"Have I ever been to California?"* "Yes, many times, I used to live there and brought you to my house at least once a year." *"I don't remember that,"* she maintained with the sweet innocence of a child.

The conversation always turned to her grandchildren, her parents', her brother and sisters' and all the places she lived. Mom sought knowledge and understanding. The heavy bag of thoughts would eventually overwhelm her memory causing Mom to collapse in tears---often slapping her head with an open hand, or banging it against the table. *"Why can't I remember?"* I quickly closed the books and let the moment pass in silence, no sense discussing Alzheimer's again.

* * *

I started considering adult daycare. For some reason, I forgot about the program, first brought to my attention by the memory facility counselor in California. I don't know why I thought adult daycare was unique to that facility. I still didn't fully comprehend the adult care industry, except assisted living, whose advertising on television now appeared ubiquitous.

Rather than in-home care, I decided Mom would benefit more by interaction with other humans. She needed activity and stimulation. Mom's disease hadn't progressed to the point where she's unapproachable, as long as it's in a controlled environment with familiar faces.

After several visits to nearby facilities, we settled on Nevada Adult Day Health Care Centers. While it wasn't a total memory care facility, several of those who attended suffered some form of dementia. Plus, daycare twice a week fit our budget, which unfortunately still mattered at this early stage of our adjustment.

Three months later, I felt like I'd finally given Mom a life. I woke her that first morning, telling her we were going for breakfast. If I'd told her the truth, she would rebel, not wanting to go anywhere without me. She dressed quickly. The physiological need for food proved a powerful motivator for action and usurped any loss of memory.

We arrived at the front door when I got a serious case of the nerves. "Was I making the right decision?" "Would she hate this place?" I pushed my feet forward despite my sudden apprehension.

A cool blast of air hit our faces as we entered the facility. The outside temperature had already hit ninety degrees at 8 a.m. Mom and I remarked in unison, "that feels good." Our remark broke the tension of the moment for me, Mom still not realizing why we were there in the first place.

The facility was a beehive of activity as caregivers and recipients scurried about in a controlled frenzy. We were greeted at the door, Mom by name. "Hi Anita," one of them said. "Let's go get some breakfast. Do you want some hot tea?" The care provider softly held Mom's hand and guided her to a table. I slipped out quietly. Wow, just like when I dropped my son off at daycare twenty-five years ago. They would distract him to provide me an escape route.

That first day was one of pure torture, not for Mom, for me. If daycare failed I'd need another plan. I had no idea what that plan would look like. I needed a distraction, so my girlfriend and me had an early lunch, followed by a movie, our first time alone in three months. I remember little of our date, my mind so consumed with Mom's welfare.

I picked her up around 3 p.m., anxious to get a read on her day. As we drove home, she asked, *"What is that place we just came from?"* Huh, you remember, I thought to myself. Instead of answering her question, I answered a question with a question, "why do you ask?" *"I don't know any of those people. You know I don't like to go places where I don't know anybody."* I let silence fill the car, allowing the hum of the air conditioner to carry the moment. Two blocks later, her memory of the days events had been wiped clean.

Mom went back the following week for two days. One foot in front of the other I kept reminding myself. I entered the facility that third day to take her home, when I noticed one of the attendants teaching her to ride a stationary bike. She loved the attention and seemed game, so I let the moment play out. After peddling for a few minutes she let out a cry of joy, happy she met the challenge. At that moment, I knew I made the right decision.

Four months later we're making plans for three days per week. I've been told she can dance an hour nonstop. Her caregivers have asked me on numerous occasions if Mom was a professional dancer in her past life. Each time they asked the question, I gave them a bemused look of sorts trying to make sense of their question.

I relayed the story of her dancing to Mom's best friend. She burst out with a deep hearty laugh, "Michael, we could never get Nita to dance during our clubbing days."

I guess Alzheimer's released the chorus girl within. It's the third time Mom's dancing prowess had been on display in less than a year. Who knew? Mom still doesn't sleep, but she's active, engaged, and happy when she attends daycare.

* * *

I took my concerns about lack of sleep to her doctor fearful she would injure herself, if her body didn't shutdown for a few hours. She was already on Donepezil, the generic form of Aricept. Donepezil improves the function of nerve cells in the brain for mild to moderate dementia caused by Alzheimer's. Even after four months, I couldn't tell if the drug worked. All I could see was continued cerebral decline. I stuck with the drug thinking maybe it slowed the progression of the disease. How do you measure the slowing of a degenerative disease that you physically can't see?

Mom had also been prescribed Namenda a few months prior in graduated doses, starting at 7MG, working our way up to 28MG daily. In layman's terms, Namenda reduces the action of chemicals in the brain that may contribute to the symptoms of Alzheimer's.

Once Mom reached 21MG, the drowsiness became so pronounced she couldn't function---unable to stand, or eat without assistance. She had difficulty raising the fork to her mouth, nodding off once nearly stabbing herself in the eye. I decided to stick with the program, thinking her body would adjust. After a month, I had enough, and removed Namenda from her regimen. It took a few days for the body to expel the drug from her system, but Mom looked, felt, and behaved better.

I shared my concerns with the doctor, both of us agreeing, no Namenda. We were all in full experimental mode, so I had no problem trying Namenda. I would do anything to slow down the ravages of this disease; it just wasn't the right approach for Mom. Everyone reacts differently to a drug. Hopefully, it will help someone else.

To combat the sleep issue, doctor's wanted to try Trazodone. It was selected because of its non-addictive qualities. Typically used to treat depressive disorders, its also used to help people relax. We started at 50MG before bedtime---two weeks later, nothing. We increased the dosage to 100MG and noticed a slight change. While she didn't sleep, I noticed it relaxed her. The constant pacing before her scheduled bedtime receded somewhat. We could safely give her a higher dose, but I decided to settle for relaxation.

A new body of research suggests lack of sleep, or waking frequently during the night, actually increases the risk of those already predisposed with Alzheimer's. Those of us in the western world are so consumed with our careers, we think nothing of little, or, interrupted sleep.

According to Rudolph Tanzi, a Harvard University neuroscientist, and one of the world's leading researchers on Alzheimer's, everyone needs to *"cycle into the deepest stage of sleep after REM, several times every night, because it's then, and only then that you stop making amyloid and clear out the plaque and other debris from the brain."* It's those amyloids and plaques researchers pinpoint as culprits for increased risk of Alzheimer's. You can read the rest of Tanzi's comments in the October 2016 issue of *AARP Bulletin*, on page 44.

Thinking back, Mom was never one to sleep more than five hours. Plaques form 15 to 20 years before there are any cognitive symptoms, says Tanzi. So get more sleep---seven to eight hours would be about right.

* * *

Mom's relationship with Rusty took on added significance as her condition worsened. She fully expects him to answer when she asks questions, angered at times when he doesn't respond using the English language. Rusty, loyal to a fault, seldom leaves her side, even when she chastises him in a tone of voice, I'm certain he recognizes as not to endearing.

"Why aren't you talking to me?" "Are you okay shrimp?" she asks no fewer than a dozen times daily, often, a dozen times within an hour. If Rusty turns his head sideways, *"Are you okay shrimp?"* If he didn't clean his plate, *"Are you okay shrimp?"* If he gets up to stretch his legs, *"Are you okay shrimp?"* Each time she asks that question I want to scream. I feel sorry for Rusty, but Mom is doing her best to show she cares for her little buddy and has few options to express herself, or remember she asked the question seconds before.

Temperatures in Las Vegas were now well into the triple digits, topping out at 115 degrees. The heat didn't abate before 10 p.m., and even then, it hovered around 100 degrees. Mom loves sitting on the balcony before bedtime. No amount of hard or soft sell could keep her off that balcony. After five minutes, Mom returned to the cool comfort of an air-conditioned house, complaining of the heat, only to return after five minutes forgetting she just left the balcony.

Unfortunately, poor Rusty followed her every step for the first few months. No amount of cold-water consumption can cool a fury animal's body temperature in such oppressive heat.

I thought Mom would unintentionally kill him, so we tried to discourage her, "Mom it's 115 degrees outside." "Mom it's blistering hot, you could get heatstroke" "Mom you're going to kill Rusty if you keep taking him outside, its too hot."

Mom had no reference point for numbers or temperature any longer. Reminding her it was 115 meant nothing. Even when I took her to daycare, she subconsciously reached for a coat not understanding it was summer in Las Vegas.

Rusty realized if he kept following her, he would suffer. So, he started to protest, mildly of course, by staying inside when she opened that door. When she forced him outdoors, Rusty immediately announced his displeasure. Mom misidentified his reasons for barking, claiming he was annoyed by the neighbors. Poor Rusty lay exhausted on the floor, tongue hanging from his mouth.

I tried one more idea. "Mom you are going to kill Rusty." I grabbed a handful of his thick fur. "See how thick this is? Stop taking him outside." Then I grabbed her skin and made her grab Rusty's simultaneously to prove a point. Nothing worked. All I could do was manipulate her sensibilities and compassion, or pray fall arrived soon.

As a test, I tracked Mom's trips to the balcony. An hour and nine trips later I quit counting, but the trips continued from morning to early evening with Rusty on her heels.

* * *

Mom's compulsive repetitive behavior is so annoying earphones and loud music have become my defense. *"Has Rusty eaten?"* is a question I get about twenty times a day. I turn up the volume so loud I risk ruptured eardrums to get relief from that and other redundant questions.

By far the most annoying of Mom's fixations outside of food, is her continuing weird paranoia with a bathroom. No matter the circumstances, in public or private, if Mom sees the words bathroom or restroom, it's off to the toilet, even if she went a second before. It's ironic that once severe stage Alzheimer's arrives, she could become incontinent, and we will wish for the days she paraded back and forth to the toilet.

Simultaneous to her compulsiveness, she has become even more child-like if that's possible. In public, she holds my giant hand in the gentlest way, and if frightened will squeeze with considerable strength. We have silly conversations, her laughing at my pedestrian grade school jokes.

At home, I'd scream at some politician on television for saying something outrageous, and she would burst into laughter, as if she understood, or maybe it was my salty language that elicited her response.

She would often ask if I would consider moving near a beach, an ode to Atlantic City. I mentioned us possibly moving to California. "Mom they have beaches in California." The resulting smile on her face is priceless.

Then she'd hesitate and look at me, the child within on full display, *"Do I get to go?"* "Of course you get to go," further cementing our being together in her head. I learned to cherish these brief interludes of warmth, knowing full well it could change faster than a freak thunderstorm.

Nothing could ever replace a beach in Mom's mind, yet her most powerful memory of recent visits to the water lasted until the point we left the shoreline. I make frequent trips to Southern California for business or Mom's medical exams, each time taking her to the beach. Mom walks several miles from the Santa Monica Pier to Venice Beach and back. The wooden blanks of the pier remind her of the Boardwalk in Atlantic City.

She loved the sights and sounds of crashing waves, beach volleyball, families riding bikes, well-trained dogs walking with their owners, and those playing basketball near Muscle Beach. Mom didn't miss a single detail.

By the time we opened the car door to leave, the beach had been consigned to oblivion. I learned to settle for small victories, but it still hurt that I couldn't provide lasting joy.

CHAPTER ELEVEN

The Day Mom Forgot

Two months after arrival --- It was an unseasonably warm day for early April, 84 degrees, and not a cloud in the sky. Humidity lingered in the high single digits like most every other day in Las Vegas, with a slight breeze---just enough to provide comfort and hazy air quality as dirt from the desert floor swirled from one barren piece of land to the next.

The mental transition from her house to ours is still a work in progress. It certainly hasn't been a smooth process. I feel for Mom, but I have to play the hand I am dealt until I could arrange for a new game.

We just finished our Sunday brunch with my girlfriend and her family, and retired to their backyard, me sipping a glass of red wine, Mom a bottle of water. Five adults in all sat quietly, not much in the way of conversation, save for brief interludes of presidential politics as the primaries rapidly approached. Mom understood nothing, completely oblivious to the discussion in her midst. I'd look at her on occasion to see if she had anything to offer. She just shrugged her shoulders and went back to whatever occupied her mind, if anything.

The trees swayed back and forth. A hummingbird, wings fluttering at blinding speed, appeared, disappeared, and reappeared, putting on a wonderful show.

After an hour, we excused ourselves and left for home, on our way out the door, as usual, we were loaded with enough leftovers to last nearly a week. We said our goodbyes, piled into the car, and started the fifteen-minute journey.

The view from the car is spectacular. Mansions and smaller Mediterranean style homes surrounded the hilly golf courses. Golf carts, legal to be driven on the roads here, dotted the landscape. From atop the hill we could see the expanse of the valley from the Spring Mountains to the Las Vegas Strip and beyond.

A steady stream of planes silhouetted against a beautiful blue sky are landing or taking off from nearby McCarran Airport. The ride home, is a peaceful one. The sights of the day captured our collective imaginations.

Once home, we greeted Rusty, tossed our shoes aside, refrigerated the leftovers and turned on the television---my girlfriend and me in the living room, Mom in her bedroom.

Thirty minutes later Mom appeared, clutching her stomach once again. "*My stomach is bloating, I've got to put something in my stomach,"* she moaned, in a deep husky voice, gasping for air. "Mom you just ate two pieces of chicken, two helpings of sweet potatoes, rice and beans, a piece of cake, and two slices of tiramisu. Mom, your body is digesting the food you just ate." *"I don't remember any of that."*

Mom retreated to her room, reluctantly at first. She settled into a comfortable easy chair to deal with the discomfort of digestion when I brought her a Lifesaver---the faux antacid. Moment's later she reappeared just as Rusty started eating his food. *"That's good pumpkin, eat your dinner."*

I could tell Mom wanted to talk. We muted the television and asked if she needed anything. The conversation started innocently enough. *"Don't I have any family?"* She'd been on a journey of discovery for the better part of a week, desperately trying to connect the dots of her fuzzy past.

Like the dozen previous times Mom asked about family, I grabbed the photo albums to provide a reference point and familiarity. We started discussing all the family she had and where they lived. I, once again, decided to conduct my own informal memory test to better gauge where this conversation was headed.

"How many kids do you have?" *"I think three."* "Do you know their names?" She rattled off three names just like she'd done before, but those weren't her kids, they were her brother and two sisters'.

My girlfriend asked, "Anita, who is that," pointing at me? Her reaction, the Alzheimer's Process Stare. She turned her head from side to side, first looking at me, then my girlfriend, then back to me. It was a crushing blow; one I was unprepared to accept. I looked away ever so briefly.

The day I warned Mom about a few weeks back just announced its arrival, only she didn't remember my prophecy. The sucker punch to my gut landed hard and heavy. Nothing prepares you for that punch, it just has to land, do its damage, and hope you remain upright until the immediate pain subsides.

Without telling Mom about our relationship, we showed her the most celebrated picture in the Bennett household. It is a black and white photo of me at about ten months old; dressed in a suit and tie, my expressive eyes wide and engaged, my curly locks on full display. It is beloved by everyone in our family. I used that photo on the front cover of my previous book. Mom had multiple copies of that photo throughout her house. My grandparents' displayed it in their home. Both my sisters' had it in theirs, even my son commented about that particular photo more times than I can count. Mom smiled at the sight of the picture. *"That's my son."*

I went through every picture in the photo album that had something to do with me from first grade through high school graduation---class photos, award ceremonies, newspaper clippings where I'd been featured, important family photos featuring me, her only son and confidant.

I held some of the photos next to my face searching her eyes, in an attempt to trigger a distant thread of recognition. Her brain couldn't make the connection between the version of the son touching her hand, and those photos.

From age 12, forward, I didn't exist. For the few pictures of my teenage years she did recognize, Mom repeated, *"that's my son,"* not once understanding those old photos and me were the same person.

My girlfriend finally pointed at me, "Anita that's your son, that's Michael, the same person in that baby picture." I showed Mom the photo of me on the front cover of my book. Her reaction, one of disbelief, *"you're kidding, that's you?"* Then she called me by her brother's name, a mistake she made occasionally over the phone, but never in person. My girlfriend touched Mom's other hand, "no that's Michael." Once again she looked at me and addressed me as her brother.

From that moment on, I realized my relationship with Mom, at least in her eyes, changed from son to care provider, or maybe just a roommate. My girlfriend looked at me, full of empathy, sadness crowding her heart, offering a touching apology in a quiet, sweet voice. I'd been wounded. I bit my lip to conceal the hurt. I knew this day would come, I just didn't think so soon. Like everything else with this sinister disease, my own mind thought I had more time.

Hearing the *Family Feud* on her television, I escorted Mom to her chair, and just like she'd done many times previously, she passed by the photos of her parents', looked at me proudly and said, *"that's my mom and dad.*" I nodded my head, acknowledging her comment, and quickly retreated.

How does one process a mother who no longer recognizes her son? This is not a movie. No hero is going to swoop in and magically restore Mom's memory. I felt empty inside---a deep void of nothingness that could never be filled by another person.

The one person I'd spent my entire life not wanting to disappoint had vanished, yet she is still very much physically present. I seldom made a move without asking myself, "What would Mom do?" even if she knew absolutely nothing about the subject. Mom has a keen moral compass that often froze me in my tracks on those rare occasions when I contemplated crossing the boundaries of acceptable behavior.

No longer would I confide my deepest darkest secrets to her care. We had a relationship that I trusted---revealing secrets about myself most sons wouldn't dare share with their mother. Mom and I were different, a byproduct of our younger days dealing with a husband and father suffering from PTSD. Dad and I could never converse or share intimate details of our lives like mom and me.

Mom played both mother and father during large portions of my youth. At some point in life, earlier than most families would consider normal, our roles reversed, me playing the elder statesman. It occurred so seamlessly, neither of us noticed, and now, it would be imperative that I seize control.

Despite Mom's absence of memory, I could still feel the bond, the love evident in how she spoke to me during her more lucid moments. It was small victory in which I'd been forced to stake my claim.

It took a few days for me to accept, albeit with profound sadness, our new dynamic. In a way, I felt liberated, free for the first time to focus on Mom's care without worry about what she thought of my decision-making.

I always felt somewhat handicapped when it came to providing for Mom. I still sought her approval even when my better judgment told me I'd made the right decision.

Sending Mom to Nevada Adult Day Healthcare Centers was one such decision that came about once she forgot I was her son.

I'm now planning Mom's future without reservation. While I still haven't made final decisions, the cloud of my own indecision has disappeared.

And to the woman I have spent my entire life idolizing, I will provide for you no matter what. I don't have all the answers yet, but I'm confident they will come. I Love You.

Michael!

CHAPTER TWELVE

Family

Since Mom's arrival, I discovered other members of my family, had suffered, or, are suffering from Alzheimer's. Some were blood relatives, others, related through marriage---all women, all on Mom's side of the family.

I wonder how vulnerable my sisters' and first cousins are to this insidious disease. The percentage of those at risk for Alzheimer's increases significantly if a family member has the disease---especially a direct lineage, mom to daughter. Through discussions with family, several are worried they too, might one day succumb to the ravages of Alzheimer's.

My cousins' and me started to exchange notes, support, words of encouragement and understanding. Some grew up with the disease as part of their daily lives caring for an elderly loved one, others, like my immediate family were newcomers, and needed all the advice we could get.

We've now surpassed our one-year anniversary of unintended exile from normalcy, to this new norm. The death of Mom's mind continues at a steady pace. My obsession now is with the future, expectantly waiting for the other shoe to drop---the day I can no longer care for the woman who brought me into this world.

I continue to struggle with the emotional detachment necessary to make good decisions. It's dawned on me that I need to redefine the meaning of emotional detachment, to maybe love attachment. Through love, I can do what's right for Mom, no matter the difficulty of such decisions. I must be aware not to allow my heart alone to decide. Each time I've allowed my heart, singularly, to make a determination; it's been the wrong choice.

When I rely on the rational part of my brain, it seldom fails. I can't fix her, I know that, I can only provide comfort, a comfort that goes unrecognized, and that's okay.

When I feel an emotional crisis of confidence coming on, I deliberately delay heart wrenching decisions, for days if necessary, depending on what's needed, pushing valiantly against the sentimental thumping of my heart.

Even Rusty has started to withdraw, preferring, at times to spend hours with me to avoid Mom's constant badgering. Her frequent angry, but non-violent outbursts aimed at Rusty for his inability to understand her commands, or accede to her demands, frightens him. Yet, at the end of the day, like me at times, he usually goes limping back to her side seeking ways to please the one love of his little life.

Mass confusion, paranoia, agitation, pacing and delusions have exacerbated. The list of items she's now fearful of includes the security lights from the apartment complex across the street. Mom's adamant those lights, clearly visible from our balcony, are new. For months she ran inside at dusk thinking those lights were some alien space ship about to descend on our doorstep.

Vouchers we've received from Helping Hands of Las Vegas and the Alzheimer's Association has allowed us to increase Mom's adult daycare attendance to three times a week. The only downside to the increased activity as far as I can tell, is her heightened state of confusion once she arrives home. It takes a good hour to familiarize herself with her surroundings. Despite Rusty's presence, Mom explores her bedroom like she's entered it for the first time.

* * *

My fiancé and I have had two date nights in nine months. Unfortunately, that first night ended with me contracting a serious case of food poison that left me bedridden for days.

The day after Thanksgiving was our second. I was admittedly nervous. It had taken me months to decide leaving Mom for a few hours in the evening is doable. I retained some residual apprehension from the day police arrived on Mom's doorstep ten months earlier. I just couldn't allow Mom to be cared for by a stranger, no matter how qualified they appeared on paper. Our first date back in April, Karen entertained Mom. This time it would be a sitter.

I'd read about all the adult sitter services offered by professional organizations in Las Vegas, but Mom, is a different creature. As sweet as she is, strangers have no place in her surroundings. It took Mom weeks to get comfortable with daycare.

Fortunately, I stumbled across a sitter acceptable to both Mom and me. The sitter was no stranger; it's one of the ladies from daycare. I've observed their interaction on numerous occasions. She brings out the best in Mom, laughing and joking more than I've seen in years. Humor always seems to work with Mom. If it weren't for Alzheimer's they could easily be good friends.

Our evening out with friends couldn't have gone better, a much-needed distraction from the monotony that had become our lives. My girlfriend actually appeared more concerned about Mom's welfare than me, rushing to get home as soon as the meal ended. We arrived to a very happy mother.

* * *

Mom's quarterly evaluations at the Cleveland Clinic are like sucker punches to the gut. Each visit serves as a harsh reminder of the inevitable. Mom, on the other hand, is completely unaware of the reasons for these visits. That's probably a good thing.

Outside of things committed to deep memory, such as her birth date or Atlantic City, it's all gone. The meaning of time, gone; remembering she has children, gone; identifying animals, familiar foods, places she's lived, my name---all unidentifiable as brain death continues.

Mom can sit for hours, doing nothing in particular and be perfectly content, no matter how much I try to engage her in activity.

The medications designed to slow down cognitive decline appear useless. All I see is deterioration. I've taken Mom off Donepezil without consulting her doctor and noticed no discernable change in behavior or cognition.

I've changed the times I administer Trazodone and increased the dosage in consultation with her doctors, it's helping in spurts. On occasion, maybe once a month, Mom will dose off for a quick nap during daytime hours. Those naps last less than fifteen minutes.

Most evenings she sleeps less than two hours. On the rare night she manages more than a few hours, the sleep is so deep she wets the bed, forcing me to restrict water intake after 7 p.m. We have no way of knowing when a deep sleep will ensue.

Removing her bottle of water at night typically leads to a battle of wills. Often, she'll sneak into the bathroom and drink from the sink faucet. Her attachment to the water bottle is more pronounced than taking a stuffed animal from a child.

Gastrointestinal problems are frequent, and her reaction is dependent on her mood at the moment. We consider it a good day if she only complains once. Most days, it's no fewer than a half-dozen times.

The intersection of Alzheimer's and bloated stomach is all consuming. When she's home the constant "uh, uh, uh, uh, uh, uh" is so annoying I want to put my fist through a wall. I can no longer discern if the habitual groans are true pain or dementia eliciting a paranoid reaction. Simply distracting Mom, more times than not, is all the relief she needs, but on those occasions where the pain is real, its frightening.

Unfortunately, providing a distraction takes hours of precious time. I've learned to ignore the "uh uh" noises unless Mom screams, and even then, it might be nothing more than a plea for attention. I'm no longer surprised how fast her stomach afflictions disappear when I arrive on the scene.

* * *

We men often take women's needs for granted. To that, I must confess guilty as charged. I've learned more about female needs and bodily functions in a year than I care to admit. I now pay attention to thinks most women take for granted---bras, panties, undergarment textures and outer garment sizes.

When Mom arrived it appeared she hadn't spent a dime on clothing since retirement. Much of her daily wear looked threadbare or discolored from constant washing. Thankfully, I had a girlfriend as equally disturbed as me about the state of Mom's wardrobe. We both set out to replenish those rags.

When my bride-to-be arrived home with Mom's new undergarments, all she could do was stare in disbelief. *"For me,"* she asked more than once before a horrified look swept across her face as she compared the new to the old. Mom recognized the Raggedy Ann look of her old underwear, the elastic stretched far beyond the boundaries of her body. The next day, she complained the new stuff was too tight. We went back to the store to buy undergarments with a looser fabric.

Over the past few months we've replaced virtually all Mom's wardrobe, deeming much of it unsalvageable, even for the needy. Knowing how Mom prided herself on outward appearance, I was truly embarrassed, we (my sisters' and me), allowed Mom's wardrobe to deteriorate.

Despite our substantial investment in new clothing, she reaches for the familiar. We've removed old, but wearable clothes, forcing her to make different choices.

* * *

Mom's two best friends from her days in Colorado had a wonderful reunion here in Las Vegas. They invited Mom. The trio reminisced for hours, while Mom sat and listened, smiling at the appropriate times. They all know of Mom's condition and made sure to include her, telling stories of the wonderful times they'd shared.

Mom remembered none of it, but took great delight in knowing she'd contributed to their happiness.

As Thanksgiving came and went, it hurt me deeply that the only persons to call Mom that day were my uncle and his beautiful family, and Mom's best friend. I desperately wanted my sisters' to call, sad for Mom when the phone didn't ring. While a call from family is only remembered in the moment it occurs, it's rewarding for me to watch Mom laugh and smile. Thankfully, they called on her birthday and Christmas less than a month later.

It's been nearly six months since Mom asked, "Do I have any family?" Mentioning the names of my sisters' or her grandchildren is greeted with silence. The pictures I've put in her room to remind her of family are nothing more than pieces of furniture to be walked around. Mom has more of an affinity with the daycare personnel than anyone except my girlfriend and me.

We enjoyed a Thanksgiving meal with my girlfriend and her extended family and friends, eighteen in all. Mom, as usual didn't say much, but she enjoyed the festive atmosphere, eating more than I'd observed in awhile, all while dressed in a new outfit we purchased over the summer and held for just such an occasion.

* * *

We took Mom to a Christmas light display at the Las Vegas Motor Speedway, a driving tour through a tunnel of lights and other festive decorations. While the rest of us were expressing our pleasure at the bright scenery, Mom remained stoic, her eyes barely registering the moment. Not once did she turn her head or make a comment. I asked a few questions trying to gauge her enjoyment. She didn't respond.

Her reaction to those lights reflects a now constant theme in her life. Mom simply doesn't respond to unknown stimuli, and if known the odds are fifty/fifty she'll have no reaction

* * *

Today marks the one-year anniversary since Mom's arrival on February 23, 2016. It's been a trying twelve months. Our collective frustrations have gotten the better of us at times, me suppressing my emotions as best I can to let others vent. That goes against all the advice I have received exhorting me to take care of myself.

To release the tension, I have returned to the gym, often for two hours. The benefit, my weight and health have all returned to normal.

On days its not too hot outside, my girlfriend and I go on walks of three to five miles, stopping for breakfast, or a cup of coffee. Often Rusty is with us when Mom's at daycare, providing him some much needed exercise.

Recently, Mom has resorted to peeing in the trashcan again. Just this week, she's wet the bed and used the can three times. We are in complete child treatment mode.

At bedtime its, "Anita go to the bathroom." I no longer ask if she has to go, I make her go.

I've also toyed with the idea of putting a portable motion detector in her room that emits an alarm to a receiving unit on my nightstand. The moment her feet hit the floor I will be awakened. Costs for such a device ranges from $80 to $250.

* * *

I've returned to work with a new sense of urgency; the need to care for Mom and my need for self-fulfillment are powerful motivators.

When business takes me away from town, I previously drove, or took the bus to California (Mom won't fly), so Mandi could watch Mom while I'm away. If my sister is unavailable, I cancel the trip, or have my fiancé care for Mom without me, which I consider a completely unfair burden for her to bear. The trips to California add at least a day to the front and back end of my journey, not to mention the expense.

In May, I'm taking my first out of town trip in six months. For someone who works in travel and tourism, is a public speaker, and toils away behind the scenes in the entertainment industry, that's an eternity.

I've stumbled across a new care model, at least new to me, to assist in caring for Mom. I first heard of group homes about six months ago, when I complained to Mom's nurse at the Cleveland Clinic about the cost of assisted living. The nurse asked if I'd investigated group homes. I'd never heard of them. I was told they were much less expensive than assisted living and more intimate in terms of the ratio of patients to care providers.

Well, low and behold, within thirty days of that conversation, without any effort from me, a group home option presented itself, by a licensed care provider who had been in my orbit for nearly a year.

After careful consideration, I've decided to have Mom stay at a group home, also referred to as Residential Care Homes, for my upcoming trip. It helps to have a sister who lives in town in case of emergencies. It's infinitely more affordable than assisted living.

Since my interview with the first group home provider, I've interviewed another, and made the painful decision that some time this calendar year, Mom will permanently move to a group home.

The one I've selected has experience with Alzheimer's patients, all the appropriate licensing, and one of the owners is a registered nurse. This is the single most difficult decision of my life, but one that will benefit Mom in the long run, as her needs are rapidly approaching a point where I'll no longer be able to care for her with the class and dignity she deserves.

My work life has become more important than ever for another reason. I'm determined not to have my son bear the burden of my senior care when that day comes. For that I must get back to work.

While I don't want to underestimate her love attachment to me, even if she doesn't remember who I am, I must do better by my mother.

Sadly, the group home does not allow residents to have dogs, which means separating Mom and Rusty, despite my best efforts to keep them together. I cried when I made that decision. I never wanted to separate them, not only for Mom's sake, but Rusty's as well. Honestly, I too became attached to Rusty, considering him more my dog than Mom's. This hurts.

Rusty always had a home with my sister back in his old house. My sister Karen, the one I affectionately call the dog whisperer, has offered more than once to care for Rusty. He'll feel right at home, if he can overcome what I'm certain will be a shock for a few days.

* * *

Like everything else in a profit-driven health care system, our success and eventual care options was totally predicated on money. Sadly, too many senior citizens are falling through the cracks of quality care as those in Washington D.C., and state capitols, play games with potential affordable care options that often mean the difference between life and death. We owe our seniors respect and better treatment than political posturing that often has us in full retreat, as opposed to advancing the twin causes of affordable care and research.

For any politician who cares to read this book, the collective horrific experiences of Alzheimer's victims is real and shouldn't be trifled with through petty bickering, empty rhetoric and broken promises. The time to act has long since passed---disaster is imminent.

EPILOGUE

The Alzheimer's train is roaring down the track, picking up speed every few weeks. At some point along its journey, severe Alzheimer's will arrive at the station. The conductor's rate so variable, its' hard to predict when the train will get to our stop, but it is coming. Many studies suggest the severe stage is often the longest, others, the moderate stage. Regardless of which stage hangs around the longest, the train will once again continue its journey towards the final stop, death.

Alzheimer's sufferers and caregivers who went before Mom left a trail of evidence difficult to ignore---financial angst aside.

When will Mom become incontinent? I shudder at the thought of what that entails---wet and soiled bed sheets, disposable diapers, smelly clothes, and more. It's all a function of aging compounded by a dreadful disease.

The ability to walk, sit, and talk could become seriously compromised. The inability to communicate could render her unable to tell us if she is in pain. That pain might be a hallucination.

Mom already suffers a lack of awareness and decades of lost memories, both a hallmark of severe Alzheimer's. Everything she experiences, good and bad, is now a new adventure that lasts no more than a few seconds.

Many Alzheimer's victims also suffer other chronic illnesses. In Mom's case its gastrointestinal.

She could have difficulty swallowing, something she already suffers from in mild form due to issues with her stomach and hyperthyroidism. Some Alzheimer's sufferers forget how to eat, the simple act of raising a fork or spoon to their mouths.

By far the most serious of all severe Alzheimer's related problems is pneumonia. Pneumonia is the most frequent cause of death in Alzheimer's patients.

If one is fortunate to survive pneumonia, death usually comes when the brain can no longer control the body and organs, hence the definition, death caused by complications from Alzheimer's.

How many of these symptoms will afflict Mom and when will they start? Will her decline be gradual or abrupt? There are so many unanswerable questions.

Mom's been with me over a year now. Compared to the day she arrived, my mother is almost unrecognizable and worsening by the day. Yet, physically, we've observed little change. It's a recipe for the Alzheimer's trap---the mind tearing the physical into shreds before its physical manifestation are observable.

Will Mom be part of that small percentage of individuals, who live beyond the eight-year threshold from diagnosis? We simply do not know and neither does anyone else. All I can hope for is that the conductor will slow the Alzheimer's train long enough to allow her to squeeze a few more enjoyable moments out of life.

Alzheimer's & Service Dogs

As you've probably gathered from reading our story, Rusty is not a trained therapy dog. He came about his love for my mother organically. Their eight-year relationship is a blessing, the timing of their union so perfect. Rusty's love is unconditional. Rusty doesn't pass judgment; and the best part much to Mom's chagrin at times, he doesn't talk back.

Mom directs most of her energy and interaction towards Rusty, in ways she could never do with me. Rain or shine, this little guy is her world. If she's gone for a second, when she returns, it's the happiest moment in both their lives, a reunion I've witnessed hundreds of times over the years. When Mom has a panic attack or throws one of her tantrums, its Rusty to the rescue.

Rusty never retreats. Mom suffered a severe leg cramp, and rather than run, or cower in fear at her screams for help, Rusty jumps on her lap to protect her from harm forcing me to remove him temporarily to provide care.

I'm not here to recommend introducing a new pet into the lives of an Alzheimer's patient. I'm not trained on the matter, but I've read several stories stressing the possible benefits of a pet. Those benefits include: lower blood pressure and heart rate, less anxiety, agitation, irritability, depression or loneliness. Some memory care facilities bring in pets for weekly visits.

If you already have a pet, try with every once of your being to keep them together. The bond might be so strong separating the two could complicate matters. Obviously someone needs to provide all appropriate care for our furry little friends, a task Mom relished, but can no longer perform adequately.

A few of the traditional assisted care facilities accept animals, but it was up to the owner to provide direct care, or pay for a service. I've inquired with a few memory care facilities about pets. Their rules are all over the map, leaning towards no.

"Are you ok shrimp?" "Are you ok pumpkin?" "Do you need to go out?" "Do you want something to eat?" "Do you want to sit outside? "Do you want some water?" These questions fly from Mom's lips no fewer than a half-dozen times an hour. The repetition is truly annoying for the uninitiated. Admittedly, it took me months to adjust, and it still bothers me at times, especially when she forces him outside during high heat warnings.

It's widely known by those with pets, dogs have an innate ability to feel for those they're close to. Rusty has shown that ability better than I could have predicted. I've found myself taking cues from Rusty as regards to Mom's feelings and emotions.

* * *

Despite their bond, as mentioned in the last chapter, I've made the painful, but necessary decision to place mom in Residential Home Care later this year. It was a decision I made, just a few weeks before releasing this book, forcing me to add this final section. Her advancing condition and my need to get back to work requires a solution, that, while I realize is a prudent one, leaves me racked with guilt.

It's been twelve days since Rusty's departure. Mom hasn't complained yet, but knows something isn't quite right. Her advancing disease has allowed her to accept the consequences, something I couldn't imagine a year ago.

Additionally, I could no longer justify risking Rusty's health. Mom unintentionally injured him a few times, in her attempts to do too much, once a trip to the vet for pain medication. With summer rapidly approaching, I'm thankful Mom won't force little Rusty outdoors in triple digit temperatures.

Rusty returned to the home he shared with Mom for eight years; the one my sister is renting from Mom. Karen takes Rusty and her other dog for walks several times a week. Rusty has a backyard where he roams freely, and gets to live the life of a dog. He's active and happy. I visit often, and know he's in good hands. I think I miss him more than Mom.

WHAT YOU SHOULD KNOW

What exactly is Alzheimer's and why should you care? I hope to answer both of these questions and more below.

In a story entitled *The Alzheimer's Laboratory*, the CBS program *60 Minutes* summed up Alzheimer's this way:

> *"An Alzheimer's diagnosis is essentially a prescription for a slow descent into oblivion, inexorable loss of the memories, spatial skills, and ability to think that made us who we are."*

Alzheimer's is named after Dr. Alois Alzheimer, a German physician, who presented a case to a medical meeting of a 51-year-old woman who suffered a rare brain disorder. After performing a brain autopsy, he identified the plaques and tangles that characterize the disease that now bears his name. The year was 1906. As of 2016, Alzheimer's is the sixth leading cause of death in the United States.

To better understand Alzheimer's we must first define dementia. Dementia is a general term for a decline in mental ability severe enough to interfere with daily life. Memory loss is one example. The most common type of dementia is Alzheimer's, which accounts for sixty to eighty percent of all dementia cases.

Dementia is caused by damage to brain cells. This damage interferes with the ability of brain cells to communicate with each other. When brain cells cannot communicate normally, thinking, behavior, and feelings can be affected.

Alzheimer's itself, is a progressive disease. Symptoms usually develop slowly and get worse over time, becoming severe enough to interfere with daily tasks, up to, and including, speech and bodily functions. Alzheimer's is ultimately fatal.

Despite decades of experiments and testing, scientists have yet to discover a cure, although several drugs have been approved to slow the progression.

Scientists believe the plaques and tangles synonymous with this disease develop more than a decade before symptoms begin. Currently, no test exists that would identify who among us might get the disease.

The myth that the Alzheimer's form of dementia is part of the normal aging process is patently false. Up to five percent of those diagnosed with Alzheimer's have what is known as early onset---symptoms that can appear in an individual before age 65.

About the time I started this book, legendary University of Tennessee women's basketball coach Pat Summitt lost her life to this terrible disease. She was just 64 and had been diagnosed with early onset several years earlier, forcing her into premature retirement.

Scientists have discovered a small fraction of eventual Alzheimer's sufferers, carry a gene mutation where it's a near certainty the carrier will get Alzheimer's, but again, one doesn't need to carry the gene to get the disease. In fact, most Alzheimer's victims don't have that specific gene mutation. For those who do carry the mutated gene, symptoms have been known to arise in the mid thirties.

Pardon me for the clinical explanation, but it's important, and I promise I'll keep it brief. A healthy human brain has about 100 billion neurons, each with long branching extensions. These extensions enable individual neurons to form connections with other neurons. These connections are called synapses. Information flows in tiny bursts of chemicals that are released by one neuron and detected by a receiving neuron. The brain contains 100 trillion synapses. They allow signals to travel rapidly through the brain's neuronal circuits creating the cellular basis of memories, thoughts, sensations, emotions, movements, and skills. That wasn't so bad was it?

You'll often hear two terms associated with the brain in Alzheimer's patients---plaques and tangles. Plaques or the more scientific name, beta-amyloid plaques are proteins outside the neuron. Tangles or tau-tangles, are proteins that form inside the neurons. It's the accumulation of plaques and the abnormal accumulation of the protein tau scientists believe contribute to the development of Alzheimer's. What causes these abnormalities I'll leave that to the scientific community to explain.

Plaques interfere with the neuron-to-neuron communication at the synapses. Tangles block the transport of nutrients and other essential molecules inside the neurons. Both are believed to contribute to cell death. The brains of people with advanced Alzheimer's show dramatic shrinkage from cell loss and widespread debris from dead and dying neurons. It was this horrifying image of Mom's MRI results that left me gasping for air.

You'll often hear about the stages of Alzheimer's. It's typically divided into three broad stages, but I've seen studies and reports referencing seven stages. For our purposes, I'll stick to the three broad stages.

Mild Alzheimer's, or early-stage, might be imperceptible to the uninitiated. A person still has the ability to function independently. They may still drive a car like my mother did, and participate in social activities. Despite this, the person may feel as if he or she is having memory lapses, such as forgetting familiar words or the location of everyday objects. Mom certainly felt this way, complaining often that she couldn't remember things, or her memory was fuzzy. Her concerns were easy for me to dismiss at the time, thinking it more a function of age. It wasn't until diagnosis a few years later that I realized Mom had already suffered through the early stages of the disease.

Moderate Alzheimer's, or middle-stage, is typically the longest stage, according to some, although, I've read research that suggests stage three is the longest. Stage two can last for many years. This is Mom's current stage, and based on my unscientific observations, she's been in this stage for at least two years. Damage to nerve cells in the brain can make it difficult to express thoughts and perform routine tasks.

Alzheimer's usually destroys short-term memories first. Those memories are stored in the hippocampus region of the brain. Most days, Mom doesn't remember what she did five minutes ago. She cannot follow the arc of a sitcom or remember what she read in a book just a second before.

Mom's forgotten most of her personal history, dating back sixty years. She has periodic bouts of moodiness that have worsened over time combined with a fear and paranoia that has her crouching in the corner of her room until some perceived danger has passed.

Mom doesn't know the day of the week or the time of day. Numbers in reference to standard measurements we all take for granted mean nothing. If I tell Mom its 100 degrees outdoors it means nothing. "Do I need a coat," she'll often ask, even if I'm dressed in shorts and a tank top with sandals. I've tried to train Mom to observe what I'm wearing to provide her a clue of the daily temperature, but Alzheimer's makes that next to im-possible.

Decision-making is difficult and practically non-existent for her. Mom could stare at her closet for hours deciding what to wear, even though we've reduced her selections to a combination of five shirts and three pants. Her dressier clothes hang in our closet for special occasions.

Other symptoms of this stage could include; wandering, becoming lost, trouble controlling bladder and bowels, delusions, repetitive behaviors, and other symptoms you've read about earlier in this book.

The third, and final stage, is severe Alzheimer's, often referred to as late-stage. As the name implies, every one of the previous stages is magnified. People can live years in a state of morbidity before death. The longevity of this stage varies in each individual, but it's this stage that routinely requires full-time, around-the-clock care.

Late-stage Alzheimer's is where the sufferer will lose the ability to respond to their environment, communications skills become severely compromised, patients are likely to experience periods of, or total incontinence, become vulnerable to infections, especially pneumonia, and may be unable to walk, sit, or swallow.

Why should you care? That's easy. While one in nine people age 65 and older has dementia, sixty to eighty percent of those have the Alzheimer's form. By age 85, nearly one in three persons have dementia. We are all going to age, and if you're unprepared, like we were, the consequences are devastating.

Risks factors increase exponentially for those who have a parent, brother, sister, or child with the illness. If more than one person in a family suffered from Alzheimer's, the risk factors increase even further.

Research has shown that groups at higher risk for vascular disease, Latinos and African Americans in particular, may also be at greater risk for developing Alzheimer's.

Of the 5.4 million Americans with the disease, nearly two-thirds are women. Why, is still being determined.

To learn more about this disease, there is a study available for download on the Alzheimer's Association website entitled, *2016 Alzheimer's Disease Facts and Figures*. This report is update annually.

Care & Costs

Of all the things I've learned about Alzheimer's to date, care costs proved more unpredictable than memory loss; the cost so exorbitant it nearly destroyed my eight-digit calculator. Whether its memory care, simple assisted living, in-home care, nursing homes, whatever the venue, with the possible exception of group homes, it's all too expensive for the average family.

Alzheimer's can easily devour an entire life's savings, long-term care insurance, home equity, a pension, social security, financial assistance of family, and the limited financial resources available through various organizations, such as the Alzheimer's Association, and still go looking for more to eat.

If ruining the finances of the sufferer isn't bad enough, caregivers, usually a spouse or their children, have been financially decimated as well. According to the *2016 Alzheimer's Disease Facts and Figures* report, us caregivers contribute between $1,000 and $100,000 of our own money annually to the cost of care. With the average life expectancy of an Alzheimer's sufferer after diagnosis at four to eight years, those dollars add up quickly. Some sufferers live as long as twenty years.

We are at the four year anniversary of Mom's diagnosis, and if I use family DNA as a guide, she will easily survive longer than eight years, assuming the destruction of her synapses doesn't accelerate faster than what I've already observed.

Our exploration of care options started with traditional assisted living, not realizing at the time, the need for memory care was imminent. In Las Vegas, Mom's retirement and social security income pushed the boundaries of her monthly financial obligations in a standard assisted living environment---that which doesn't require memory support. We would have to liquidate Mom of every financial obligation she currently has, including her mortgage to afford that basic level of care.

We can't sell her home or take out an equity line of credit. Thanks to the avarice of Wall Street, her home is $40,000 underwater just to match the loan payout. So our choices are walking away from the home, or marketing it as a rental. We chose the later and found a tenant immediately, my sister.

Traditional assisted living without the bells and whistles carries a monthly price tag of approximately $3,500 in Las Vegas. Then comes the addons. If you have a pet, some places charged an additional $250 deposit plus a small monthly fee, even if the resident is perfectly capable of caring for their own animal.

Need prescription drugs administered, $200 a month. Need transportation to and from the doctor or a local store, add another $75 to $150. Oh, I forgot to mention, most places have an initial deposit requirement. In Las Vegas it averages $2,500.

So what does the basic service get you? It gets you a bed, possibly with a roommate, three meals daily plus snacks, basic cable service, access to a nurse 24-hours a day, maybe laundry service and weekly room cleaning (some places charge extra for laundry and weekly room cleaning) and daily activities for the residents.

In Mom's case, simple assisted living, even now, wouldn't be a high enough level of care---she needs memory care now.

One of the least expensive memory places I found started at $4,500 a month with a roommate. By the time we finished with additional expenses, that figure soared to $6,000. I can't verify the veracity of the following statement, but some have told us they pay as much as $9,000 a month for residential memory care. For Las Vegas, that seems extremely high, but for places like California, not so much.

Knowing I'd planned to move back to Southern California, I checked a memory care only live-in facility and found their base price started at $7,800 a month. With extra fees, our costs would actually exceed that $9,000 by a few pennies.

A little simple math revealed I would be one of those caregivers giving closer to $100,000 annually for Mom's needs if I kept her near me in California. Mom's monthly pension combined with social security tips the scales at $3,500 a month. If we wound up at this particular facility, I'd need to contribute $66,000 annually of my own income. Needless to say, like many middle class families, I don't have that kind of money. If Mom lives another six years, which I fully expect, I'd spend nearly $400,000 to provide for her care.

Simply moving Mom to one of Southern California's inland communities would reduce the bite out of my wallet to a mere $24,000 annually.

After much research, I discovered lower cost of living areas typically had more affordable prices. I can't speak to the quality of care based on these cost differences; I'm simply reporting what I've discovered.

Once I started making inquiries into memory care, my phone rang non-stop for weeks as intake coordinators attempted to sell me on the virtues of their facilities. To me, it felt somewhat disconcerting that Mom's future had been reduced to a sales call. I have no doubt those who called were well intentioned. The callers were polite and professional, but if you're sensitive to nuance like I am, even the hint of sales tactics is offensive. Only one person tried the stereotypical car salesman approach, and he's probably still licking his wounds.

Despite my reservations, I visited several residential memory care facilities and realized they provide a valuable service that shouldn't be underestimated, if that's where your loved one eventually winds up.

Before I knew much about the Devil's Disease, each time I visited a memory care place, the patients appeared to be in a trance, unable to communicate. Stupid me didn't realize at the time, that the ability to communicate is compromised in severe Alzheimer's patients. When combined with the fear and paranoia often associated with strangers in their environment, this behavior is perfectly normal.

When I evaluated Alzheimer's care facilities, I looked for things like resident to provider ratio. Is the staff trained to handle Alzheimer's sufferers, or simply money mills? I observed everything, and I typically did this without Mom.

Another long-term care solution that recently came to my attention is group home care, sometimes referred to as Residential Care Homes (RCH) or board and care, you read about in the last chapter. It's defined as a home where a small number of unrelated people in need of care, support, or supervision can live together. Several people have mentioned this to me as an alternative to more expensive care options noted above.

The cost is typically between $2,500 and $6,000 a month, a significant savings over assisted living memory care, and much more intimate. An in-home 24-hour nurse would cost three to five times the amount of an RCH.

Most group homes have state licensing requirements that must be met before opening this type of business. Most are concerned with zoning requirements, not specifics of what happens inside the home. It will include things like no signage on the property advertising the home as an RCH, or obtaining the appropriate business license. Does the home have appropriate locks and alarms in place to protect not only the home, but prevent Alzheimer's patients from wandering off. Be forewarned, some state regulatory requirements are more developed than others. One of the best I've found to date is California.

Also, digging up information can be down right frustrating, as the infrastructure is still under development in many states.

In addition, the licensing of the individuals charged with your loved ones care; are they trained nurses, etc., varies from state to state. And lastly, Alzheimer's specific care training seems to be lacking across the board. Several states I contacted had no such training program for caregivers. In California, when I started this book, a bill had been introduced to include Alzheimer's specific training into the required course work for any facility, group home, or otherwise, wanting to work with Alzheimer's sufferers.

Adult Day Care in Las Vegas starts at $75. In California's more populated areas those prices can climb to $125 or more, daily.

Adult daycare, like so many other forms of care, is often marketed as respite care for the care provider---but the benefits to Mom, when she started, and even now, appear more profound. The interaction with a warm and friendly staff has revealed her long dormant sense of humor in ways I couldn't have imagined. She smiles more, and jokes with the staff, often at my expense; on the days she remembers I'm her son. The games, the exercise, and interaction with others have made daycare worth the price of admission.

There are dozens of in-home care providers, willing to come to us, but I specifically sought an environment where she interacted with a group.

Despite my requirement that a provider has training in Alzheimer's care, Nevada doesn't appear to have very many, if any, who have met this requirement, in large measure because Alzheimer's specific courses aren't offered. Many care agencies claim they have training with dementia patients, but what's that mean? Did they learn only after they took on a sufferer? Did they take a specific course? Are those courses certified? I've asked around, and most have told me there's no official certification course, something I find quite odd given the length and severity of this disease.

An organization I vetted, but decided not to pursue at this time is Visiting Angels. They provide a 24-hour in home service split by two care providers into two 12-hour shifts. They use the same two nurses to provide stability and recognition. Costs range from $17 to $20 an hour depending upon how you use the program---at

$17 an hour that works out to $408 a day, or $2,856 a week.

Nothing we've found to date will alleviate the extreme financial burden on families. As baby boomers age, with longer life expectancies, experts predict an explosion in diagnosed cases. The resultant financial strain placed upon sufferers, care providers, and governments isn't unique to the United States, but those costs are better managed in advanced nations without profit-driven care models.

A number of European countries, even with their generous national health insurance programs, are drowning in both new Alzheimer's patients and debt driven by care costs. It's been reported that some European countries send sufferers to less expensive locales in Europe and across the planet to cope.

I've spoken to several individuals in Las Vegas who sent their loved ones to the Philippines at a fraction of the cost. Las Vegas has a large Filipino American population, but many non-Filipinos consider this a viable option.

Another destination of choice is Thailand. Early reports suggest those who've availed themselves of these locales like the level of care provided and its lower cost. Many spouses of the dementia patient have relocated to stay near their loved one. For those who can handle the cultural change, this might be a worthwhile solution.

The day of reckoning is here. While it might take decades to find a cure for the underlying disease, given the paltry amount of research dollars allocated, the urgency for affordable care options can't wait any longer. This disease could easily wipe out entire health care systems placing a drag on economies worldwide, even robust ones like the United States.

Alternative Quality Care Advances

I am particularly enamored by an idea dubbed "Dementia Village" by CNN. This Dutch, cutting-edge elderly care facility is the most innovative approach I've read to date. This isolated village just outside of Amsterdam is roughly the size of ten football fields. Residents are given a quality of life that appears normal.

Dementia Village is set up like its own small town complete with a town square, theater, garden, and post office. Individual residences within the village are tailored to lifestyles with many design furnishings dating back to the 1950s, 1960s or the 2000s. The reason is simple; their experts believe it might put the patient in contact with a familiar look and feel from their past, attaching itself to those memories that might still remain. I wonder if I could get an Atlantic City room? There are cameras everywhere, and many of the plain-clothed people walking the streets are actually the nurses and specialists charged with their care.

Would the economies of scale, given the rapid growth in diagnosed cases allow something like this to thrive in the United States---highly doubtful. But what I like about the Dutch approach is the focus on living, not death, and their out-of-the-box perspective to this global crisis.

The best part of this solution might be the costs. As of 2014, it cost $9,000 a month for residents, but the most any single person pays is $3,600. The government subsidizes the difference. I have to emphasize, this is not a perfect solution, but its far more advanced than anything I've seen to date. There is a second Dementia Village planned for Rome, Italy. You can learn more at dementiavillage.com.

Financial Resources

Alzheimer's, as you've read, requires substantial amounts of capital for the sufferer and/or family care provider to survive. It's the single most expensive disease to manage and so costly, its driven otherwise financially healthy families into bankruptcy. No single disease should ever wipe out a life's worth of savings and investments, but here we are, and sadly, there's no end in sight. Below are options for the less fortunate, financially.

Medicare and health insurance is an absolute must. This is the one area where my mother had a distinct advantage over so many others. Mom has both Medicare and a secondary insurance provider, where the premium for that secondary provider is deducted from her pension. Even with such great insurance, we paid thousands in out-of-pocket expenses to handle the myriad needs of an aging person, all compounded by

Alzheimer's. There is no direct Alzheimer's assistance through Medicare, but it does cover our visits to the Luo Ruvo Brain Institute as part of normal health coverage. Medicare does provide skilled nursing and therapy after a hospital stay, but no more.

Social Security offers no direct coverage for Alzheimer's. You either have social security benefits, or you don't. The Social Security Administration, thanks to the advocacy of the Alzheimer's Association and others, has added early onset/younger onset Alzheimer's to the list of conditions under its Compassionate Allowance Initiative, giving those with the disease expedited access to Social Security Disability Insurance and Supplemental Security Income.

Home equity might be the biggest source of funds available for those who own a house. Every person I've spoken to, and every website I researched; all recommended taping into home equity. That wasn't an option for us, but for those with substantial equity and the means to pay your loan, or, sell outright and pocket the cash for care, it's a great resource.

Personal savings, what little Mom had, was wiped out within two years of diagnosis. She had four emergency room visits the first year alone. The bills piled up, but if it weren't for her health insurance, it could have been a lot worse. Additionally, maintenance on her house not covered by today's home insurance, combined with ridiculous deductibles for those repairs the policy actually covered, exacerbated our situation ten fold.

Medicaid is for people with very low incomes and assets. In Nevada, the threshold is approximately $2,100 in monthly income and less than $2,000 in assets. Mom didn't qualify. Even if a person qualifies, they are required to pay a portion of their own care, and that percentage of cost varies from one state to the next.

Veteran's assistance is available for our nation's finest and their surviving spouse. Everywhere I turned, those in the know asked, "Is your mom a veteran, or the surviving spouse of a veteran?" Surviving spouses can receive up to $1,140 a month. I couldn't believe my luck. My spirits jumped through the roof at my discovery, only to find out my mother doesn't qualify. Those benefits, combine with Mom's income would have put us on the threshold of a lower cost memory care facility.

A group called **American Veterans Aid** is easily the most caring group of people I spoke to throughout the entire process of my search for capital. Unfortunately, three questions later, we were disqualified, because my dad remarried about ten years before his passing, after being single for decades. Mom would get nothing for her sacrifice. I was embarrassed at my reaction, so anxious I was to find Mom, and by extension me, financial relief. I have nothing against Dad's widow. We are close to this day, but my mother earned those benefits, and it's a colossal slap in the face that her sacrifice would go unrewarded. I hope, at some point, they change this requirement.

Long Term Care Insurance (LTCI) I must admit is an area where I plead ignorance. I'd never heard of LTCI until Mom started suffering. The pros and cons of this insurance, at least for now appears to tip towards the cons. Long-term care covers a whole host of services from home care, to adult daycare, and residential care in an assisted living facility or nursing home. It's designed for people who can't take care of themselves for extended periods of time.

To even qualify for this policy, you'd better be in good health at the time of application. Remember, insurers are in the business of making money.

Sadly, according to an article I read in AARP entitled *Understanding Long-Term Care Insurance*, this coverage is not cheap. Annual premiums are in the thousands of dollars and can shoot up without warning. "The LTCI landscape is confusing, unpredictable, and clearly unregulated," according to the story. "Two deterrents in particular – high cost and the yearly use it or lose it nature of the product" makes this unpalatable for most.

I did a cryptic computation of monthly premiums using a Genworth Financial Calculator based on my age, 58, at a daily maximum benefit of $250, for four years. My annual premium would be $3,475 in Nevada.

These policies can be extremely complicated and come with riders, such as, inflation protection, that add to the cost along with something called elimination protection.

Check out the website **American Association for Long-Term Care Insurance** (aaltci.org) for information on the industry. This site is a professional organization for the industry and policy providers; so make sure you read between the lines to protect your self-interests--- Caveat Emptor---Buyer Beware.

Vouchers allowed us to land on our feet. We were awarded one from the local Alzheimer's Association chapter in Las Vegas for $500 and a supplemental one about six months later. These vouchers are only good once per fiscal year. We used ours to pay for mom's adult day health care.

We've recently received a second voucher through the **Helping Hands of Vegas Valley** worth $1,000 on an annual basis. Trust me, every little bit helps.

Another organization I've heard great things about, but haven't utilized yet, is **Hilarity for Charity**. This organization, founded by writer Laura Miller Rogen, and her husband, actor Seth Rogen has provided vouchers totaling 56,000 hours for in-home care.

Support Groups

This might be one of the most neglected resources available to both the Alzheimer's suffer and their families. When doctors at the Luo Ruvo Brain Institute first mentioned support groups to me, I must admit, not only was I skeptical, I dismissed it outright. For those of you who don't have the resources at your disposal that I have, I highly recommend using one. Remember to "take care of yourself."

I don't want to sound like a hypocrite, since I've never availed myself of their services, but you need support. I'm fortunate, or unfortunate depending upon ones perspective, to have numerous family members and friends who've dealt with Alzheimer's. They paved the way to my education and are a valuable resource that I can tap into at a moment's notice. They've allowed me to vent my frustration, provide emotional support, and make recommendations on how to handle Mom. Without them, I'd be lost.

In Las Vegas, there are no fewer than a dozen support groups, some very specialized for Veteran's, Spanish Speakers, and Early Stage Alzheimer's that prepare you for the road ahead. Others are just general groups that discuss a little bit of everything. All are typically free. You can find a list of support groups through your local Alzheimer's Association chapter.

Trained facilitators lead these groups. Participants share information and ideas. They provide a platform for best practices that build coping skills that you'll need to survive. Trust me when I tell you, you will need all the help you can get.

MedicAlert® + Safe Return®

Wandering is a huge risk with Alzheimer's. Mom currently doesn't wander, but I'm not oblivious to the fact that could change at a moment's notice. I've read far too many stories of Alzheimer's sufferers leaving the friendly confines of their homes, completely lost.

In one recent case, police shot and killed a dementia sufferer after neighbors reported a burglar. When officers arrived, fearful the man had a weapon in his pocket, officers shot him because he couldn't understand their commands to remove a hand from his pocket. Only later did officers discovery his hand was wrapped around a crucifix. The MedicAlert + Safe Return is a nationwide identification and education program that mobilizes first responders should an individual become lost. There is an initial enrollment fee, but scholarships are available to eligible families to assist with this cost.

Communication

Communicating with an Alzheimer's patient is like learning a new language in patience and understanding. People with dementia typically have difficulty express-ing thoughts and emotions. They also have more trouble understanding others.

When Mom moved in, I communicated with her like I always had, expecting her to pick up on every nuance and inflection in my voice. I used vocabulary and phrases like everything was right in the world.

After a week of struggles, I realized Mom didn't truly comprehend half of what came out of my mouth, to polite to express her displeasure. Thanks to advice from family, friends, and the Alzheimer's Association, I changed my approach. It took me awhile to adjust, but now it's second nature.

We've all spoken to someone, but had our eyes riveted on a computer screen or television, never once turning our head to acknowledge their physical presence. I worked hard to change this behavior. Now, when Mom speaks, I stop what I'm doing, look her in the eye, and when appropriate, respond, hanging on her every word. This simple jester made all the difference in the world.

I've always thought of myself as a mind reader. My son and I often joked about how we were always ten steps ahead of those communicating with us, frustrated waiting for them to catch up. When Mom has trouble communicating, I usually know where she's going, but I've trained myself to wait. When Mom truly gets lost in thought, I will complete her sentence or nudge her back on track in a non-demeaning manner. For this to work, I have to be engaged and vested in the conversation. Mom usually responds with a broad grin, relieved she didn't have to remember where she was going. "Yeah, you know what I meant," she'd say with a grin.

I avoid being critical of Mom at all cost and seldom correct her, regardless of who is right or wrong. Fortunately, the relationship we have was always based on respect and good communication. Outside of our argument about her unwillingness to make late life decisions, our communication couldn't be better. The only difference between then and now, I've become even more sensitive to refraining from criticism.

It might sound silly on the surface, but feelings matter more than facts. I always know when Mom is serious. She often addresses me as "Mister Michael" when she wants something done, or needs my attention. I pay rapt attention to her tone of voice. You can never predict what's truly important to an Alzheimer's sufferer.

I avoid arguing. I thought this would be easy given the relationship Mom and I enjoyed, but it proved to be the most difficult challenge. I've learned to dodge and deflect if necessary to avoid an argument I have no way of winning. Mom's gastrointestinal problems and obsession with food, as you read earlier, have led to some ugly confrontations.

It took months to change my behavior. I've even resorted to telling a small lie, or two, like giving her a Lifesaver and telling her it's an antacid so she won't overeat. I hate doing this, but the result of the argument is ten times worse. I know the gastrointestinal attacks will go away in less than thirty minutes.

Here's a quick list of tips and techniques I've used for better communication with mom. You'll find these and others on the Alzheimer's Association website.

- Call her by name---it works for my girlfriend, for me it's mom
- Use short simple words and sentences
- Speak slowly and clearly
- Give one-step directions
- Ask one question at a time
- Patiently wait for a response

- Repeat information or questions as often as necessary
- Turn questions into answers
- Avoid confusing expressions
- Avoid vague statements
- Emphasize key words
- Give visual clues
- Avoid quizzing
- Give simple explanations
- Write things down
- Treat the person with dignity and respect
- Be aware of your tone of voice
- Pay special attention to body language

I've used some combination of each of these recommendations on a daily basis. For Mom, some carry more weight than others. For example, Mom is extremely sensitive to tone of voice. Speaking with the slightest hint of anger is typically greeted in kind.

Short declarative sentences without jargon and twenty-first century colloquialisms are a must. None of those hip phrases today's millennial and Gen-X folks use makes sense to Mom. Even my baby boomer colloquialisms she grew up hearing no longer resonate.

Repeat---repeat---repeat. I've grown sick and tired of constantly repeating myself, but repeat you must. The reason I now give Mom one task at a time, it's easier for her to stay focused. "Mom, put your shoes on." I say nothing more until the shoes are on.

While none of the above makes sense to the uninitiated, it makes perfect sense to those of us providing care. I learned much of this through trial and error and the school of hard knocks before realizing I had so many resources at my disposal. At the end of this book is a list of those resources.

Pressure

As a group, we must pressure lawmakers, insurance companies, research institutes, governments, and others to fund more research, and create a more cost-effective and comprehensive care plan. The combined dollar cost of lost work hours and sharply rising care expenses in America is nearly half-a-trillion dollars, that's trillion with a "T," annually. That's nearly a quarter of California's entire economy, the world's sixth largest. Alzheimer's care inflation will continue to increase, both as the number of cases rise, and the simple laws of economics as companies look to maximize their profits. This is one disease that can't sustain business as usual.

Spending just $489 million on research is a crime. If you think the United States Congress is paying attention, take a look at Seth Rogen's testimony back in 2014. Pay particular attention to around 5:15 and note the number of empty chairs.

Youtube.com/watch?v=hvdbHSGWags

The crisis is already here. The time for action long since passed. We have a habit in America of being reactive as opposed to proactive, and I'm afraid we've already started down this slippery slope. This needs our attention now. Our collective ignorance, my family included, should not be repeated by those of you currently unaffected. There's a high probability this disease will touch your lives, directly, or indirectly in the years ahead.

RESOURCES

Alzheimer's Association – alz.org
Alzheimer's Foundation of America – alzfdn.org
American Veteran's Aid – americanveteransaid.com
Dementia Village – dementiavillage.com
Helping Hands of Vegas Valley – hhovv.org
Hilarity for Charity – hilarityforcharity.org
Lou Ruvo Center for Brain Health – Cleveland Clinic
Clevelandclinic.org
National Institutes of Health – nih.gov
Visiting Angels – visitingangels.com
aPlace For Mom – aplaceformom.com
National Alzheimer's Disease Awareness Month –
November
Medicaid – check local state department of aging
Support Groups, Assisted Living, In-Home Nursing
Check with local Alzheimer's organization

ABOUT THE AUTHOR

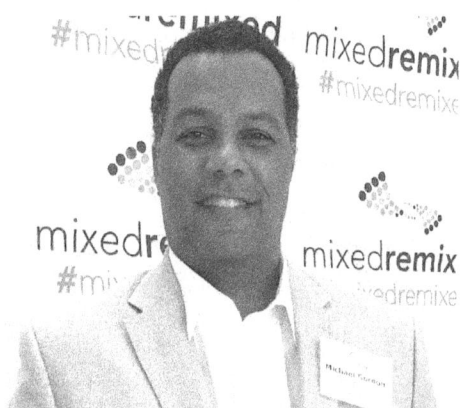

Author, actor, host, speaker, producer, travel expert, and entrepreneur Michael Gordon Bennett, is founder and CEO of Bennett Global Entertainment (BGE) a media, motion picture and television production company. His many professional accomplishments include: television and radio news producer, advertising executive, marketer, magazine writer and blogger at The Huffington Post He's also a film, commercial and television producer.

Bennett's first book, the critically-acclaimed *7-10 Split: My Journey as America's Whitest Black Kid* is a boldly written memoir of his life as a military brat; his participation in the greatest social and cultural experiment in American history, and how that experience led to intense confusion about his racial identity, and moments of heart wrenching isolation.

Bennett was appointed to BrandUSA as part of the Travel Promotion Act signed into law by President Barack Obama. He currently serves on the board of directors for the Travel Professionals of Color. He is a graduate of California State University, Northridge with a BA in Journalism and an Air Force veteran. To learn more about Michael, go to his website: www.michaelgordonbennett.com.

Bennett is a much sought after speaker, host and lecturer. To inquire about possible appearances please send an email to:

contact@michaelgordonbennett.com

or

call 702-608-4589